"The Book of Inspiring & Thought Provoking **CANCER** Quotes."

compiled by

Scott duPont

**"The Book of
Inspiring & Thought Provoking CANCER Quotes."**

Compiled by Scott duPont

Released and published by:

Nemours Publishing
c/o Nemours Marketing, Inc.
7531 Azurebrook Court
Winter Park, FL 32792
Tel: (407) 738 - 1608

ISBN # 13:

U.S.	$9.99
Canada	$12.99

Other Books in the "Inspiring Quotes" Series

Buttered Popcorn for Your Soul

Even <u>MORE</u> Inspiring Show Business Quotes

Even <u>MORE</u> of the World's Most Inspiring Quotes

*The Book of
Inspiring & Thought Provoking HEALTH Quotes*

The Greatest Book of Inspiring Quotes

The Greatest Book of Inspiring Show Business Quotes

Yet Even <u>MORE</u> of the World's Most Inspiring Quotes

Acknowledgements

I'd personally like to thank every single contributor to this book. It's my hope that in the next few years in my travels, I'll get to thank many more of you "in person". In the event that I don't get that opportunity, please know that your work in the health, medical or fitness fields and/or your research and inspiration has already helped countless people. For the many brave souls who have dealt with cancer and came out victorious including Kris Carr, Suzanne Somers and others, you are an inspiration and role models for all of us!

I'd also like to thank my early science, biology, anatomy and physiology teachers. You hooked me at a young age and the fascination of science and later health took me on a life long journey including this book that is a privilege to share with the world! A special thanks to Dr. Robert Young, Charlotte Gerson and others for your many years of research and to people like Ty Bollinger and Tony Robbins who are educating the masses about the importance of a proper alkalinity balance, which I describe as the secret kryptonite against cancer! Special posthumous thanks to Dr. Otto Warburg and Dr. Max Gerson who are heroes to so many, and among the original pioneers in researching cancer therapies.

Thank <u>YOU</u> for getting this book. I hope that by reading a few quotes each day, you will find the strength, courage and inspiration to keep moving onward and upward!

Foreword

The idea for this particular book (in the ongoing series of "Inspiring Quotes" books) came as more family and close friends were getting diagnosed with cancer the last few years. Instead of putting together another General "Health Quotes" book (the book Dr. Oexner and I compiled was well received), the thought was to put together a new book to serve the needs of individuals who hear those three (3) dreaded words you never want to hear: "You have cancer". More than anything, cancer patients need hope, clarity, inspiration, positivity, and more information about how to proceed with a life that will never be the same. That's the mission and purpose of this new "Cancer Quotes" book. My hope is that this book will also be a comfort to the immediate family, spouses, and close friends supporting those going through the challenge.

In this book, there are controversial quotes and statements about alternative treatments to the standard protocol of chemotherapy, radiation, and surgery prescribed by oncologists and medical doctors in the established medical community. I believe ALL options should be considered, both traditional & alternative. Also included are controversial quotes about shifting away from meat and dairy products towards a plant-based diet. I felt compelled to include these as there are now tens of thousands of documented cases of cancer survivors living perfectly healthy, cancer free lives following unorthodox treatments and diets. Many are my friends and myself included as a cancer survivor. Even within the traditional medical establishment (albeit very small) there are more oncologists and doctors now admitting that many of these alternatives (treatments and diets) are working wonders and in many cases with better outcomes for patients than traditional treatments. My goal and mission with this book is to open your mind and expand your thinking, before you make any decisions. It is NOT to try to sway you to become vegetarian or forgo the advice of your oncologist (in fact it's illegal for me to give any advice). The decisions you make as a cancer patient are very personal and decisions for YOU to make alone or with the support of your loved ones and family. I'm confident that the medical experts as well as the cancer survivors who have contributed quotes to this book will expand your vision, bolster your confidence, and give you real lasting hope!

Like the "Inspiring Quotes" books in the series, this book is meant to be slowly savored and enjoyed over time. Perhaps you keep this on your coffee table or your night stand and read a few quotes when you wake up, or before you retire to motivate you. If you find a quote that resonates with you, I encourage you to follow that particular author and read his or her books, follow their blogs, join their YouTube channel, or even reach out to them for more information that can help YOUR personal journey.

Disclaimer: while our team at Nemours Publishing has done our best to insure the accuracy and proper author credit for every quote, we can't guarantee with absolute certainty in the course of history (some of the quotes are hundreds of years old), who the original author is. Also, there are several doctors (Oncologists, M.D.'s, PhD's, etc.) and other notable titles in this book whose quotes we included. We did NOT include their "titles" or letter distinctions, since some of their quotes were first written or spoken <u>before</u> they had earned those degrees. We also did not want to prejudice the other excellent quotes from health & cancer experts, nutritionists, or cancer survivors who have worked in their respective field(s) for decades and/or or beaten their diseases with flying colors, but chose not to get a post graduate or medical degree.

Remember you are not alone and a BIG part of the journey is expanding your "attitude of gratitude". If you are still alive and reading this book, you already have many things to be thankful for.

Hope you enjoy!

Scott duPont

"The majority of publications equate the effect of chemotherapy
with (tumor) response, irrespective of survival. Many oncologists
take it for granted that response to therapy prolongs survival,
an opinion which is based on a fallacy and which
is not supported by clinical studies.
To date there is no clear evidence that the treated patients,
as a whole, benefit from chemotherapy as to their quality of life."
- Ulrich Abel

"A cheerful frame of mind, reinforced by relaxation...
is the medicine that puts all ghosts of fear on the run."
- George Matthew Adams

"One of the things that came out of my own personal healing
from toxic element contamination was a renewed,
almost hyper-magnified sense of compassion
for fellow human beings."
- Mike Adams

"Today, more than 95% of all chronic disease is caused by
food choice, toxic food ingredients, nutritional deficiencies
and lack of physical exercise."
- Mike Adams

"In Russia most of the hospitals
don't have any pain medicine,
they don't have any money.
So if you're with kids with cancer,
they can have metastases to the bone;
which some say is the worst pain a human can experience.
So a mother can be in a room with a child who hasn't stopped
screaming in five months...
eighty-five percent of the time I walk in there as a clown
they'll stop screaming."
- Hunter Doherty "Patch" Adams

"Laughter releases endorphins and other natural mood elevating
and pain-killing chemicals, improves the transfer
of oxygen and nutrients to internal organs.
Laughter boosts the immune system and
helps the body fight off disease,
cancer cells as well as viral, bacterial and other infections.
Being happy is the best cure of all diseases!"
- Hunter Doherty "Patch" Adams

"The longer the shelf life, the shorter your life."
- Matt Agorist

"A positive attitude may not solve all your problems,
but it will annoy enough people to make it worth the effort."
- Herm Albright

"I am not afraid of storms for I am learning how to sail my ship."
- Louisa May Alcott

"Don't count the days, make the days count."
- Muhammad Ali

"Nuts are part of a healthy diet and
studies show those individuals who eat
nuts five times a week or more
live longer than those who don't."
- Luann Alemao

"Disease is a natural result obtained from an unnatural lifestyle."
- Richard Anderson

"Cancer affects all of us, whether you're a
daughter, mother, sister, friend, coworker, doctor, or patient."
- Jennifer Aniston

"To one who has faith, no explanation is necessary.
To one without faith, no explanation is possible."
- Thomas Aquinas

"The energy of the mind is the essence of life."
- Aristotle

"The self-indulgent man craves for all pleasant things...
and is led by his appetite to choose
these at the cost of everything else."
- Aristotle

"We are what we repeatedly do.
Excellence, then, is not an act, but a habit."
- Aristotle

"We have two options, medically and emotionally:
give up or fight like hell."
- Lance Armstrong

"God gave us the gift of life;
it is up to us to give ourselves the gift of living well."
- François-Marie Arouet (aka Voltaire)

"The art of medicine consists in amusing the patient
while nature cures the disease."
- François-Marie Arouet (aka Voltaire)

"There is not one,
but many cures for cancer available."
- Robert Atkins

"In a world of prayer, we are all equal in the sense
that each of us is a unique person,
with a unique perspective on the world,
a member of a class of one."
- Wystan Hugh Auden

"Some days there won't be a song in your heart.
Sing anyway."
- Emory Austin

"Clearly, conventional cancer treatments have an important place
in medicine and save lives. But since the 1950s,
evidence has steadily accumulated that surgery, radiation,
and chemotherapy are far less effective
than the public is being led to believe."
- Kenny Ausubel

"The life you have left is a gift. Cherish it.
Enjoy it now, to the fullest. Do what matters, now."
- Leo Babauta

"Every problem has a gift for you in its hands."
- Richard Bach

"You are never given a wish without also being given
the power to make it true."
- Richard Bach

"Nature, to be commanded, must be obeyed."
- Francis Bacon

"Sugar is very toxic to your cells.
It actually speeds up the aging process."
- Bita Badakhshaw

"Nearly 40 to 75% of the world's population
is vitamin D deficient, the deficiency and disease
that follow do not need to exist.
GrassrootsHealth was founded to eradicate
the vitamin D deficiency epidemic."
- Carole Baggerly

"I'm a vegetarian - I think there's a strong possibility,
had I not become a vegetarian,
I would not be working now.
I became a vegetarian about 25 years ago,
and I did it out of concern for animals.
But I immediately began having more energy
and feeling better."
- Bob Barker

"I think that age as a number is not nearly as important as health.
You can be in poor health and be pretty miserable at 40 or 50.
If you're in good health, you can enjoy things into your 80s."
- Bob Barker

"None of us can be free of conflict and woe.
Even the greatest men have had to accept
disappointments as their daily bread -
the art of living lies less in eliminating our troubles
than in growing with them."
- Bernard M. Baruch

"I put hibiscus flower in every cup of tea I have.
It's sweet, sexy, and cleansing."
- Mario Batali

"Protein has been intensely over-represented on the plate.
Now, the garden should be the main drag for main courses."
- Mario Batali

"Medications are palliatives.
They are not designed to cure
the degenerative diseases of the body."
- F. Batmanghelidj

"When it is dark enough, you can see the stars..."
- Charles A. Beard

"People are so afraid of authority figures
and doctors are authority figures."
- Martha Beck

"I'm a very, very healthy eater. I eat lots of fish,
lots of vegetables, lots of fruit. I don't eat junk food."
- Victoria Beckham

"If it's white, don't bite.
It's best to stay away from refined, processed foods."
- Kathy Bee

"Every tomorrow has two handles.
We can take hold of it with the handle of anxiety
or the handle of faith."
- Henry Ward Beecher

"If you want to be better than you are today,
you have to want to be healthy."
- Matt Bellace

"The next time you get upset, try writing about the event.
Make sure you write out as many details as you feel are necessary.
As you go about the rest of your day or week,
explore whether or not you feel better."
- Matt Bellace

"To be good at achieving natural highs
you have to be able to express yourself in a healthy way."
- Matt Bellace

"Age is strictly a case of mind over matter.
If you don't mind, it doesn't matter."
- Jack Benny

"Drink only non-calorie containing beverages,
the best choices being water and green tea."
- John Berardi

"Happiness is good health and a bad memory."
- Ingrid Bergman

"Time is shortening. But every day that I challenge
this cancer and survive is a victory for me."
- Ingrid Bergman

"I was raised really, really healthy,
pretty much vegetarian and a very clean lifestyle,
I don't smoke, I don't drink. I'm more addicted to
the things that make me feel good
- endorphins after working out."
- Elizabeth Berkley

"Whenever you notice your thoughts detour into attack mode,
say out loud or to yourself:
'Happiness is a choice I make'."
- Gabrielle Bernstein

"This evidence is overwhelming at this point.
You eat more plants, you eat less other stuff, you live longer."
- Mark Bittman

"The USDA is not our ally here.
We have to take matters into our own hands,
not only by advocating for a better diet for everyone
- and that's the hard part, but by improving our own.
And that happens to be quite easy.
Less meat, less junk, more plants."
- Mark Bittman

"It is now evident that plant chemicals, vitamins,
and minerals can attack cancer cells at all levels,
but at the same time have no harmful effect
on normal cells while powerfully protecting
normal cells from becoming cancer cells."
- Russell Blaylock

"90% of oncologists would not choose chemo
for themselves, their spouses or children."
- Ty Bollinger

"Chemotherapy can kill many of the cancer cells
and shrink the tumors,
but it is proven to stimulate cancer stem cells."
- Ty Bollinger

"Drugs don't cure. They mitigate symptoms but they don't cure."
- Ty Bollinger

"In 1953, the US Senate determined
that there was a conspiracy to
suppress natural cancer treatments in the US.
So it is no longer a conspiracy theory, it's a fact."
- Ty Bollinger

"There's always hope."
- Ty Bollinger

"Unfortunately most modern oncologists
don't look for the cause of the cancer.
They are only treating the symptoms."
- Ty Bollinger

"I asked. I said, 'What choices do I have?
Wait, I'm not sure if I want to take that route'.
I knew I didn't want to take that route."
- Pamela Bost

"The important part to know here is that in integrative medicines
we do have that availability of building the immune and detoxing
and that's what I would like to do.
That's what Jonathan would like to do. Jonathan is working
on getting his DVDs out there where he is
talking to the children himself and he's saying,
'We have to do this therefore,
we're going to fight like crazy to do this'."
- Pamela Bost

"Two-thirds of illnesses originate in the mind.
What the mind believes, the body manifests."
- Will Bowen

"Want an excuse to do a surgery, just do an MRI."
- Mike Boyle

"Enjoy the little things, for one day you may look back
and realize they were the big things."
- Robert Brault

"Fearlessly accept the reality; then fearlessly set
about transforming what needs to change."
- Elena Brower

"Yoga has led us not only to the beauty,
magic and majesty of our bodies,
but to the opportunities to make it right with ourselves,
and right with our families."
- Elena Brower

"For I have in fact cured my own cancer,
the original site of which was the lower bowels,
through Essiac alone."
- Charles Brusch

"Every human being is the author of his own health or disease."
- Gautama Buddha

"Holding on to anger is like grasping a hot coal with
the intent of throwing it at someone else;
you are the one who gets burned."
- Gautama Buddha

"Let us rise up and be thankful,
for if we didn't learn a lot at least we learned a little,
and if we didn't learn a little, at least we didn't get sick,
and if we got sick, at least we didn't die;
so, let us all be thankful."
- Gautama Buddha

"Peace comes from within. Do not seek it without."
- Gautama Buddha

"The secret of health for both mind and body
is not to mourn for the past,
not to worry about the future,
or not to anticipate troubles,
but to live the present moment wisely and earnestly."
- Gautama Buddha

"To keep the body in good health is a duty,
otherwise we shall not be able to
keep our mind strong and clear."
- Gautama Buddha

"Nothing in excess is good for us,
so I always make sure
to balance my hard work with
recovery, rest, good food, and play."
- Kathryn Budig

"Here is the world.
Beautiful and terrible things will happen.
Don't be afraid."
- Frederick Buechner

"A long healthy life is no accident.
It begins with good genes,
but it also depends on good habits."
- Dan Buettner

"Centenarians are still living near their children
and feel loved and the expectation to love.
Instead of being mere recipients of care,
they are contributors to the lives of their families.
They grow gardens to contribute vegetables,
they continue to cook and clean."
- Dan Buettner

"Clean water is the best longevity beverage on earth.
The Adventists believe you should drink seven glasses a day
- which can keep your arteries flowing better
and organs functioning higher.
We also found that herbal and green teas
probably have a strong longevity claim."
- Dan Buettner

"Exercise, from a public health perspective,
is an unmitigated failure.
The world's longest-lived people live in environments
that nudge them into more movement.
They don't use power tools, they do their own yard work,
they grow a garden."
- Dan Buettner

"Food is the entrance ramp for better living."
- Dan Buettner

"Have fun, be active.
Ride a bike instead of driving, for example."
- Dan Buettner

"Having a purpose and knowing exactly what your values are
will add additional years to your life."
- Dan Buettner

"I can tell you that the longest-lived are getting 95%
of their calories from plants and only 5% from animal products.
Contrary to what the Paleo or Atkins diet says,
these folks actually eat a high carb diet.
About 65% of their diet is whole grains, beans and starchy tubers.
No matter where you go, the snack of choice is nuts.
People who eat nuts live 2 - 3 years longer than non-nut eaters."
- Dan Buettner

"I think we live in a culture that relentlessly pursues comfort.
Ease is related to disease.
We shouldn't always be fleeing hardship.
Hardship also brings people together.
We should welcome it."
- Dan Buettner

"One of the big things I've learned is that there's
an advantage to regular low-intensity activity."
- Dan Buettner

"The longest lived people eat a plant-based diet.
They eat meat but only as a condiment or a celebration.
Nothing they eat has a plastic wrapper."
- Dan Buettner

"The people you surround yourself with influence your behaviors,
so choose friends who have healthy habits."
- Dan Buettner

"Walking is the only way proven to stave off
cognitive decline - it works."
- Dan Buettner

"Flowers always make people better, happier, and more helpful;
they are sunshine, food and medicine for the soul."
- Luther Burbank

"If exercise could be packaged into a pill, it would be the
single most prescribed and beneficial medicine in the nation."
- Robert Butler

"I think that in modern medicine,
the demonization of the placebo effect is ridiculous...
If we can elicit this type of response from the power of belief,
it is our ethical and fiduciary responsibility as a doctor to do so. "
- Rashid Buttar

"Our patients don't look like traditional cancer patients.
They look healthy!"
- Rashid A. Buttar

"You cannot have cancer if you have
an adequate and functioning immune system."
- Rashid A. Buttar

"I want men to know that things really do get better
- and they get better fairly rapidly.
Don't get discouraged."
- George Campbell

"Life is without meaning. You bring the meaning to it.
The meaning of life is whatever you ascribe it to be.
Being alive is the meaning."
- Joseph Campbell

"Americans love to hear good things
about their bad habits."
- T. Colin Campbell

"Casein, and very likely all animal proteins,
may be the most relevant
cancer-causing substances that we consume."
- T. Colin Campbell

"Costs have so consistently outpaced inflation that
we now spend one out of every seven dollars
the economy produces on health care."
- T. Colin Campbell

"Fact is that certain people are making an
awful lot of money today selling foods that are unhealthy.
They want you to keep eating the foods they sell,
even though doing so makes you fat,
depletes your vitality and shortens and degrades your life.
They want you docile, compliant and ignorant."
- T. Colin Campbell

"Good health is about being able to
fully enjoy the time we do have.
It is about being as functional as possible
throughout our entire lives and avoiding crippling,
painful and lengthy battles with disease.
There are many better ways to die, and to live."
- T. Colin Campbell

"I have heard one doctor call high-protein, high-fat, low-
carbohydrate diets 'make-yourself-sick' diets,
and I think that's an appropriate moniker.
You can also lose weight by undergoing chemotherapy
or starting a heroin addiction,
but I wouldn't recommend those, either."
- T. Colin Campbell

"It's never too late to start eating well.
A good diet can reverse many of those conditions as well.
In short: change the way you eat and
you can transform your health for the better."
- T. Colin Campbell

"Nutrients from animal-based foods
increased tumor development while nutrients from
plant-based foods decreased tumor development."
- T. Colin Campbell

"Other countries spend, on average, only about one-half
of what the U.S. spends per capita on health care.
Isn't it reasonable, therefore, for us to expect
our system to rank above theirs?
Unfortunately, among these twelve countries,
the U.S. system is consistently
among the worst performers."
- T. Colin Campbell

"Population studies begun forty to fifty years ago show that
when people migrate from one country to another,
they acquire the cancer rate of the country to which they move,
despite the fact their genes remain the same."
- T. Colin Campbell

"Side effects of those very same prescription drugs
are the third leading cause of death,
behind heart disease and cancer. That's right!
Prescription drugs kill more people
than traffic accidents. According to Dr. Barbara Starfield,
writing in the Journal of the American Medical Association in 2000,
'adverse effects of medications'
(from drugs that were correctly prescribed and taken)
kill 106,000 people per year.
And that doesn't include accidental overdoses."
- T. Colin Campbell

"The foods you consume can heal you faster and
more profoundly than the most expensive prescription drugs,
and more dramatically than the
most extreme surgical interventions,
with only positive side effects."
- T. Colin Campbell

"Wait until you're really sick',
could be the motto of doctors and hospitals
in the current system.
'We can do nothing for you until
your symptoms surpass the subclinical and
reveal themselves in pain, loss of function,
or a particularly worrisome test result.
Until then, keep calm and keep
eating the Standard American Diet'."
- T. Colin Campbell

"What made this project especially remarkable is that,
among the many associations that are relevant to diet and disease,
so many pointed to the same finding: people who ate the most
animal-based foods got the most chronic disease.
Even relatively small intakes of animal-based food were associated
with adverse effects. People who ate the most plant-based foods
were the healthiest and tended to avoid chronic disease."
- T. Colin Campbell

"You can't patent a recommendation to eat lots of fruits,
vegetables, nuts, seeds, and whole grains.
So there's no incentive for industry to invest in such research
and no incentive for researchers to study and validate such claims."
- T. Colin Campbell

"The easiest diet is, you know, eat vegetables, eat fresh food.
Just a really sensible healthy diet like you read about all the time."
- Drew Carey

"I think I have to remain eternally oblivious to age.
Honestly, when you put a number on it yourself,
it's just like, Why? Why do that?"
- Mariah Carey

"Most of the important things in the world
have been accomplished by people who have kept on trying
when there seemed to be no hope at all."
- Dale Carnegie

"He who has health, has hope,
and he who has hope, has everything."
- Thomas Carlyle

"Change your plate. Change your fate."
- Kris Carr

"If you don't think your anxiety, depression, sadness
and stress impact your physical health, think again.
All of these emotions trigger
chemical reactions in your body,
which can lead to inflammation
and a weakened immune system.
Learn how to cope, sweet friend.
There will always be dark days."
- Kris Carr

"If you really want to turn your health around,
start juicing today."
- Kris Carr

"I knew when I was diagnosed with cancer
the only thing I could control was what I ate,
what I drank and what I would think."
- Kris Carr

"Processed foods cause inflammation,
a source of most chronic illnesses as well as stress."
- Kris Carr

"There's a great metaphor that one of my doctors uses:
If a fish is swimming in a dirty tank and it gets sick,
do you take it to the vet and amputate the fin?
No, you clean the water. So, I cleaned up my system.
By eating organic raw greens, nuts and healthy fats,
I am flooding my body with enzymes, vitamins and oxygen."
- Kris Carr

"Whether you're reaching for one of your favorite cookbooks
or just winging it, do your best to keep a well-stocked arsenal
of healthy ingredients at your disposal. At the very least,
you'll always be ready to whip up a green juice or smoothie."
- Kris Carr

"The mind controls so much of the body.
We are much more than flesh and blood;
we are complex systems.
Patients do better when they have faith
that they're going to do better.
That's why I always tell my patients and their families
not to neglect their prayers.
There's nobody I don't say that to."
- Ben Carson

"We should be concerned not only about
the health of individual patients,
but also the health of our entire society."
- Ben Carson

"Never continue in a job you don't enjoy.
If you're happy in what you're doing,
you'll like yourself, you'll have inner peace.
And if you have that, along with physical health,
you will have had more success than
you could possibly have imagined."
- Johnny Carson

"Emotions; both positive & negative,
move as electric energies
through the nervous system,
affecting the entire organism.
The nervous system carries impulses
& instructions to every cell in the body.
Positive & negative thoughts could therefore
physically alter each cell's functioning.
Worry & fear is the greatest foe to a healthy physical body."
- Edgar Caynce

"The body's cells must act in concert to sustain good health."
- Edgar Caynce

"I encourage patients and families to continually
look for the miracle but don't try to define it.
In other words, if the only miracle we are looking for is the big one
- the one where there is a miraculous cure, then we will most likely
miss the other miracles that are unfolding
before our very eyes, each and every day.
- Wayne Charlton

"I always tell my patients to eat the rainbow and
half of your plate should be colorful fruits and vegetables."
- Nalini Chilkov

"If insurance companies paid for lifestyle-management classes,
they would save huge sums of money. We need to see
that alternative medicine is now mainstream."
- Deepak Chopra

"If we are creating ourselves all the time,
then it is never too late to begin
creating the bodies we want instead
of the ones we mistakenly assume we are stuck with."
- Deepak Chopra

"I, of course meditate for two hours every morning.
It's part of my schedule;
I wake up at 4 am every day and I love it."
- Deepak Chopra

"Modern medicine, for all its advances,
knows less than 10 percent of what your body knows instinctively."
- Deepak Chopra

"Preventive medicine isn't part of a physician's everyday routine,
which is spent dispensing drugs and performing surgery."
- Deepak Chopra

"The real secret to lifelong good health
is actually the opposite:
Let your body take care of you."
- Deepak Chopra

"The way you think, the way you behave, the way you eat,
can influence your life by 30 to 50 years."
- Deepak Chopra

"Adopting a new healthier lifestyle can involve changing diet
to include more fresh fruit and vegetables
as well as increasing levels of exercise."
- Linford Christie

"Don't put off living to next week, next month,
next year or next decade.
The only time you're ever living is in this moment."
- Celestine Chua

"Attitude is a little thing that
makes a big difference."
- Winston Churchill

"Healthy citizens are the greatest asset
any country can have."
- Winston Churchill

"Never, never, never give up."
- Winston Churchill

"We shall draw from the heart of suffering itself
the means of inspiration and survival."
- Winston Churchill

"All illness comes from two causes,
PARASITES and POLLUTANTS."
- Hulda Regehr Clark

"Don't push happiness off until
you hit some future milestone.
Allow yourself to be happy in the moment.
Be happy while you are working on the task.
While you are working on building your skill set,
rather than thinking it is something you will get to
once you are good enough."
- James Clear

"Generate a system. Plan out how you will stick to your habits,
how are you going to stay passionate and focused?"
- James Clear

"If you want to eat more vegetables,
you could limit yourself to only one type of vegetable this week.
By limiting the number of choices you have to make,
it's more likely that you'll actually eat something healthy
rather than get overwhelmed trying to figure out
all of the details of the perfect diet."
- James Clear

"My work is focused on a simple idea:
I want to share practical ideas and proven research
that helps you master your habits, optimize your performance,
and take control of your health and happiness."
- James Clear

"You have to start with a version of the habit
that is incredibly easy for you.
It must be so easy that you can't say no to doing it
and so easy that it is not difficult at all in the beginning."
- James Clear

"Any family doctor will tell you
that people will stay healthier and
long-term of cost to the health system will be lower
if we have comprehensive preventive services.
You know how all of our mothers told us that an ounce
of prevention was worth a pound of cure?
Our mothers were right."
- Bill Clinton

"Despite the dedication of literally millions
of talented health care professionals,
our health care is too uncertain and too expensive,
too bureaucratic and too wasteful.
It has too much fraud and too much greed."
- Bill Clinton

"Drug companies should no longer charge
three times more for prescription drugs
made in America here in the United States
than they charge for the same drugs overseas."
- Bill Clinton

"In recent years the number of administrators
in our hospitals has grown by four times the rate
that the number of doctors has grown.
A hospital ought to be a house of healing,
not a monument to paperwork and bureaucracy."
- Bill Clinton

"Running helps me stay on an even keel
and in an optimistic frame of mind."
- Bill Clinton

"I would give up everything to have good health."
- Kurt Cobain

"Walking is magic. Can't recommend it highly enough.
I read that Plato and Aristotle did much of their
brilliant thinking together while ambulating.
The movement, the meditation, the health of the blood pumping,
and the rhythm of footsteps... this is a primal way
to connect with one's deeper self."
- Paula Cole

"I'm healthier now than I was before I had cancer."
- Lourdes Colon

"As everyone knows, cancer is pandemic
and it is growing out of control.
And we know now how to prevent cancer. I tell every patient,
it is very easy to prevent cancer,
but it is not easy to treat cancer.
So if we can all learn how to find and detect -
and now we have amazing science and technology
to figure out and prevent cancer..."
- Leigh Erin Connelly

"The blood delivers the groceries,
the lymph removes the garbage."
- Leigh Erin Connelly

"We do surgery all day long like it's no big deal.
But no, you need to prepare the patients
for two weeks for surgery, mentally and physically.
Are their nutrients good? Are they eating well?
Are they prepared to heal after surgery?
So all of my patients before we even do surgery
because sometime surgery is necessary -
I prepare them two weeks and get them nutritionally,
physically, and mentally sound to be prepared
so that surgery is easy and they can recover beautifully."
- Leigh Erin Connelly

"Other things in your life take second place."
- Sean Connery

"Don't put all your health and fitness eggs in one basket.
Work equally hard on your nutrition, exercise,
cognitive skills, and personality."
- Bret Contreras

"The power of life and death is in the tongue…
victory over cancer is a decision, not a happening."
- Francisco Contreras

"First move well, then move often."
- Gray Cook

"Moving isn't important, until you can't."
- Gray Cook

"Original humans were on their feet
for a large part of the day without leisure
or entertainment opportunities
designed around sitting in one place."
- Gray Cook

"Pain is not the problem
- it's the signal."
- Gray Cook

"Quitting unproductive practices early and
moving on to something better
is a hallmark of successful people."
- Gray Cook

"The only thing documented for depression
that does not have side effects is exercise."
- Gray Cook

"You gotta break a pattern before you can make a pattern!"
- Gray Cook

"The reason I exercise is for the quality of life I enjoy."
- Kenneth H. Cooper

"We are involved in youth testing internationally.
We want to try to prove without a shadow of a doubt
the relationship between physical fitness and health,
not just physical fitness and ability to perform."
- Kenneth H. Cooper

"I believe that parents need to make nutrition education
a priority in their home environment.
It's crucial for good health and longevity to instill
in your children sound eating habits from an early age."
- Cat Cora

"My true role as a practitioner is to empower and facilitate
healing that comes from within."
- Gaston Cornu-Labat

"Eating real food, reading labels, getting junk out of schools.
There are some things that can be done immediately.
But in terms of public policy we need to open up
a dialogue with well-intentioned people who are now
better aware of the issue and the whole confluence
of things that have come together to
create an environment in which this generation
will live shorter lifespans than their parents."
- Katie Couric

"How can you set dietary guidelines and
also be responsible for promoting U.S. agriculture,
especially when some of that agriculture
means unhealthy products?"
- Katie Couric

"Research shows that what works and is healthy
for adults also works well for children,
if adjusted to be age-appropriate.
Children, like adults, do not suffer from a deficiency
of white sugar, white flour, junk food, or processed foods.
A growing child as well as an adult is hurt by
junk foods and benefited by healthy foods."
- Gabriel Cousens

"Hearty laughter is a good way to jog internally
without having to go outdoors."
- Norman Cousins

"It is reasonable to expect the doctor to recognize
that science may not have all the answers to
problems of health and healing."
- Norman Cousins

"The capacity for hope is the most significant fact of life.
It provides human beings with a sense of destination
and the energy to get started."
- Norman Cousins

"The human body experiences a powerful
gravitational pull in the direction of hope.
That is why the patient's hopes
are the physician's secret weapon.
They are the hidden ingredients in any prescription."
- Norman Cousins

"Your heaviest artillery will be your will to live.
Keep that big gun going."
- Norman Cousins

"The longer I live the less confidence I have in drugs
and the greater is my confidence in the
regulation and administration of diet and regimen."
- John Redman Coxe

"More than ever,
you need to be an advocate for your health."
- Eric Cressey

"More than 10 million Americans are living with cancer,
and they demonstrate the ever-increasing possibility
of living beyond cancer."
- Sheryl Crow

"Every evening I turn my worries over to God.
He's going to be up all night anyway."
- Mary C. Crowley

"Happiness lies, first of all, in health."
- George William Curtis

"Be gone excuses."
- Chantal Dalabona

"Keep it simple.
It's the little things you do everyday
that make a world of difference in
your health & overall state of being."
- Chantal Dalabona

"When you accept the invitation
to embrace a healthier lifestyle,
a transformational shift happens.
You have just given yourself permission to
gain energy, clarity and strength by doing the things
you need to do and trusting in the process."
- Chantal Dalabona

"Your body is a beautiful gift,
the only one you have,
so how about giving it some loving."
- Chantal Dalabona

"Old age ain't no place for sissies."
- Bette Davis

"Running long and hard is an ideal antidepressant,
since it's hard to run and
feel sorry for yourself at the same time."
- Monte Davis

"Any doctor will admit... you see if you're put
on high blood pressure drugs,
they'll tell you that you'll be on them the rest of your life.
Why? Because they don't cure anything,
They only cover up the symptoms."
- Lorraine Day

"After discovering cancer,
I changed my diet completely."
- Lorraine Day

"Caffeine is an abnormal stimulant."
- Lorraine Day

"Cancer doesn't scare me anymore."
- Lorraine Day

"Diseases just don't happen."
- Lorraine Day

"Drugs and surgery is all
we were taught in medical school."
- Lorraine Day

"If people go on a vegetarian diet,
exercise on a regular basis and decrease alcohol intake,
a study done at Harvard School of Public Health
revealed that they will decrease
the incidence of cancer by 66%."
- Lorraine Day

"In medical journal articles that doctors read,
there are more pages in the medical journal of 4-color
high priced pharmaceutical ads,
then there is medical information!"
- Lorraine Day

"The body is made to heal itself."
- Lorraine Day

"We give these diseases to ourselves one day at a time
by what we eat and the way we live."
- Lorraine Day

"What we're eating is actually destroying us.
It's actually causing cancer and other diseases."
- Lorraine Day

"You cannot develop cancer unless your
immune system is suppressed."
- Lorraine Day

"We don't have to get sick as we get older."
- Aubrey de Grey

"When you look at people around the world who live past 100,
the one thing they all share in common
is a laid back happy attitude."
- Aubrey de Grey

"If you can stay on top of your health by
monitoring it and not guessing,
there is no reason to fear cancer."
- Veronique Desaulniers

"You have to be sick in order to develop cancer.
You don't get cancer and then get sick."
- Veronique Desaulniers

"Nothing matters more than your health. Healthy living is priceless.
What millionaire wouldn't pay dearly for
an extra 10 or 20 years of healthy aging?"
- Peter Diamandis

"Cancer is a word, not a sentence."
- John Diamon

"I really believe the only way to stay healthy is to eat properly,
get your rest and exercise.
If you don't exercise and do the other two,
I still don't think it's going to help you that much."
- Mike Ditka

"What 'The Quest for the Cures' gave us
and also Dr. Buttar, was hope that you can
heal naturally, that there are so many things
that I believe God has given us in the world that can
build up your immune system, can remove toxicities,
and can also just increase your vitality and your overall health.
I believe that I've experienced all of those through the
unconventional treatment that we chose and this path."
- Betsy Dix

"The power of love to change bodies is legendary,
built into folklore, common sense, and everyday experience.
Love moves the flesh, it pushes matter around.
Throughout history, 'tender loving care' has uniformly
been recognized as a valuable element in healing."
- Larry Dossey

"Cancer didn't bring me to my knees,
it brought me to my feet."
- Michael Douglas

"My mother was a P.E. teacher,
and she was kind of a fanatic
about fitness and nutrition growing up,
so it was ingrained in me at a young age.
As I get older, I'm finding out it's not about getting
all buffed up and looking good.
It's more about staying healthy and flexible."
- Josh Duhamel

"For the first 50 years of your life
the food industry is trying to make you fat.
Then, the second 50 years,
the pharmaceutical industry is
treating you for everything."
- Pierre Dukan

"I go jogging for 25 minutes every morning,
even if I'm away from home."
- Pierre Dukan

"It's been proven that fitting more activity
into your day can greatly improve your health."
- Pierre Dukan

"If you put on weight it's not by chance.
You put on weight because you eat compulsively."
- Pierre Dukan

"There is nothing unhealthy about
educating youngsters about nutrition."
- Pierre Dukan

"To be a nutritionist in France,
you must be a doctor, seven years studies,
and then three more years in nutrition."
- Pierre Dukan

"You never see a French person eating alone."
- Pierre Dukan

"Kids are killing themselves with energy drinks.
Literally, in my health seminars I show parents
the newspaper articles about
all these teenagers who've died
from drinking too many energy drinks!"
- Scott duPont

"Great health is the KEY
to every other part of your life."
- Scott duPont

"The old adage: 'Doing the same things every day and
expecting different results is the definition of insanity'.
This is especially true with your health.
The great news is a few small changes in your daily habits
and routines can lead to massive results!"
- Scott duPont

"For 99% of the people I work with, I tell them:
'There's NO excuse for not walking,
or at least moving every day'.
If it's below freezing outside, dress warm.
If you can't stand, use a walker.
If you have no legs, use your arms to push your wheelchair.
If you stop moving, you're dying!"
- Scott duPont

"More people need to realize how incredibly harmful
sugar is to all aspects of their health.
Just like the taxes now on tobacco products,
the best deterrent (and solution) will be
a tax on foods with ridiculously high sugar content."
- Scott duPont

"People think I'm excessive making a priority of
exercising every single day including Sunday & holidays,
saying I should rest.
My reasoning is exercise gives me lots of energy,
clears my head and I feel great!
Why wouldn't I want to have tons of energy
and feel great every day?"
- Scott duPont

"Unless you prioritize time EVERY DAY
for yourself & your health, things will never change.
Don't wait until tomorrow."
- Scott duPont

"We see people eating factory-farmed animals pumped full of
antibiotics, steroids & growth hormones which were in turn fed
genetically modified plants sprayed with pesticides and
grown in top soil treated with petro chemical fertilizers
and finally frozen and treated with preservatives
before being thawed & microwaved for our meals.
And we're SURPISED that almost 50%
of the U.S. population has cancer?!"
- Scott duPont

"Shifting to a low-sugar, lower carbohydrate diet
is particularly important for people looking to
lose weight or repair their metabolism,
and it seems prudent for everyone."
- John Durant

"Permit yourself at least two weeks
of 'mellow yellow' time per year.
This is time on vacation.
Vacation time and time away is critical
to restore and reenergize your spirit.
Book it in advance and don't change it!"
- Todd Durkin

"Set up your home gym so it's your sacred space.
Put up motivational quotes on the wall,
hang pictures that inspire you.
Put a few plants in there and let some natural sunlight in.
Make it a place you want to work out in,
a place where you want to go to take care of yourself."
- Todd Durkin

"Be miserable. Or motivate yourself.
Whatever has to be done,
it's always your choice."
- Wayne Dyer

"Doing what you love is the cornerstone of
having abundance in your life."
- Wayne Dyer

"It is impossible for you to be angry
and laugh at the same time.
Anger and laughter are mutually exclusive
and you have the power to choose either."
- Wayne Dyer

"It makes no sense to worry
about things you have no control over
because there's nothing you can do about them,
and why worry about things you do control?
The activity of worrying keeps you immobilized."
- Wayne Dyer

"Simply put, you believe that things
or people make you unhappy,
but this is not accurate.
You make yourself unhappy."
- Wayne Dyer

"Stop acting as if life is a rehearsal.
Live this day as if it were your last.
The past is over and gone.
The future is not guaranteed."
- Wayne Dyer

"There is no scarcity of opportunity to
make a living at what you love;
there's only scarcity of resolve
to make it happen."
- Wayne Dyer

"When you dance, your purpose is not to get to
a certain place on the floor.
It's to enjoy each step along the way."
- Wayne Dyer

"When you judge another, you do not define them,
you define yourself."
- Wayne Dyer

"The doctor of the future will no longer treat
the human frame with drugs,
but rather will cure and prevent disease with nutrition."
- Thomas Edison

"Life is like riding a bicycle.
To keep your balance, you must keep moving."
- Albert Einstein

"Look deep into nature,
and then you will understand everything better."
- Albert Einstein

"Nothing will benefit human health and increase the
chances for survival of life on earth as much as
the evolution to a vegetarian diet."
- Albert Einstein

"The greatest enemy of truth is to have faith in authority."
- Albert Einstein

"There are only two ways to live your life.
One is as though nothing is a miracle.
The other is as though everything is a miracle."
- Albert Einstein

"People need to realize that there's no such thing as a
'Lipitor deficiency' or a 'Crestor deficiency',
yet we keep taking these types of pills every day."
- Bruce Ellington

"Always do what you are afraid to do."
- Ralph Waldo Emerson

"All the pre-made sauces in a jar,
and frozen and canned vegetables,
processed meats, and cheeses which are
loaded with artificial ingredients and sodium
can get in the way of a healthy diet.
My number one advice is to eat fresh, and seasonally."
- Todd English

"It takes more than just a good looking body.
You've got to have the heart and soul to go with it."
- Epictetus

"Preach not to others what they should eat,
but eat as becomes you, and be silent."
- Epictetus

"The key is to keep company only with people who uplift you,
whose presence calls forth your best."
- Epictetus

"We are not dealing with a scientific problem.
We are dealing with a political issue."
- Samuel Epstein

"Prevention is better than cure."
- Desiderius Erasmus

"Most people focus on working OUT to lose weight,
but if you want to see results that
last a lifetime start working IN...
Change the Mind
Change the Body."
- Vanessa Esperanza

"We tend to look in the mirror and
focus on what we don't like...
If we just focus on what we do like,
we'll see more of THAT
next time we look in the mirror."
- Vanessa Esperanza

"Cholesterol is a white, waxy substance that
is not found in plants - only in animals.
It is an essential component of the membrane
that coats all our cells, and it is
the basic ingredient of sex hormones.
Our bodies need cholesterol,
and they manufacture it on their own.
We do not need to eat it.
But we do, when we consume meat, poultry, fish, and
other animal-based foods, such as dairy products and eggs.
In doing so, we take on excess amounts of the substance.
What's more, eating fat (even as added oil) causes the body
itself to manufacture excessive amounts of cholesterol,
which explains why vegetarians who eat oil, butter, cheese, milk,
ice cream, glazed doughnuts, and French pastry
develop coronary disease despite their avoidance of meat."
- Caldwell Esselstyn

"Collectively, the media; the meat, oil, and dairy industries;
most prominent chefs and cookbook authors; and our own
government are not presenting accurate advice
about the healthiest way to eat."
- Caldwell Esselstyn

"Every mouthful of oils and animal products,
including dairy foods, initiates an assault
on these (cell) membranes and,
therefore, on the cells they protect.
These foods produce a cascade of free radicals in our bodies
- especially harmful chemical substances that induce metabolic
injuries from which there is only a partial recovery.
Year after year, the effects accumulate.
And eventually, the cumulative cell injury is
great enough to become obvious,
to express itself as what physicians define as disease.
Plants and grains do not induce the deadly cascade of free radicals.
Even better, in fact, they carry an antidote.
Unlike oils and animal products,
they contain antioxidants, which help to neutralize the
free radicals and also, recent research suggests, may provide
considerable protection against cancers."
- Caldwell Esselstyn

"I believe that coronary artery disease is preventable,
and that even after it is underway,
its progress can be stopped, its insidious effects reversed.
I believe, and my work over the past twenty years has
demonstrated, that all this can be accomplished without expensive
mechanical intervention and with minimal use of drugs.
The key lies in nutrition - specifically, in abandoning the toxic
American diet and maintaining cholesterol levels well below
those historically recommended by health policy experts."
- Caldwell Esselstyn

"The best and safest thing is to keep a balance in your life,
acknowledge the great powers around us and in us.
If you can do that, and live that way, you are really a wise man."
- Euripides

"Breathe, Relax, Let Go and Allow your Life to Flow."
- Sharon Feanny

"If you want to Detox it takes 3 days to Let Go,
7 Days to Renew and
21 Days to a Whole New You!"
- Sharon Feanny

"It's not just what you put in your body,
it's also what you put ON your body that matters!"
- Sharon Feanny

"My Mantra for a healthy and happy life is
Live Fit, Live Life and
Most Importantly, Live LOVE!"
- Sharon Feanny

"Stop counting calories in your food
and start counting the vitality that
the food you are eating will give you
- that's how you lose weight!"
- Sharon Feanny

"Ultimately we know deeply that the other side
of every fear is a freedom."
- Marilyn Ferguson

"Nothing is so healing as the human touch."
- Bobby Fischer

"Go vegetable heavy.
Reverse the psychology of your plate
by making meat the side dish
and vegetables the main course."
- Bobby Flay

"I learned a long time ago that the last thing any woman
should be thinking about is being 'skinny' or 'thin.'
To me, those words imply weakness, fragility,
the inability to stand firm in a storm.
If you want to change your body, aim for 'athletic'.
An athletic body is healthy, strong, and built to thrive.
An athletic body can take many shapes."
- Lauren Fleshman

"Make your race a playground,
not a proving ground."
- Lauren Fleshman

"Elsewhere the paper notes that vegetarians and vegans
(including athletes) 'meet and exceed requirements' for protein.
And, to render the whole
'we-should-worry-about-getting-enough-protein
and therefore-eat-meat' idea even more useless,
other data suggests that excess animal protein intake is linked
with osteoporosis, kidney disease, calcium stones
in the urinary tract, and some cancers.
Despite some persistent confusion,
it is clear that vegetarians and vegans tend to
have more optimal protein consumption than omnivores."
- Jonathan Safran Foer

"Both doctors and patients often forget,
in the midst of cancer treatment,
that the aim is to get people well."
- Ann Fonfa

"I'd like to see CER and clinical studies be about
what helps people get well.
Right now we are looking for the 'active ingredient' of a food.
In my mind, it's not one ingredient, it's a food.
We can't treat food as a pharmaceutical."
- Ann Fonfa

"If someone is in treatment or just finished treatment,
they should use the help of a professional;
a nutritionist, a naturopath, an acupuncturist.
Someone who works with these issues a lot
who can look at the alternatives to
complement chemo and radiation and surgery."
- Ann Fonfa

"No matter how conservative you are medically,
there is always room for complementary therapies."
- Ann Fonfa

"Our focus is on complementary and
alternative approaches to cancer,
in the belief that many of them have
a great deal to add to this goal.
Complementary approaches like diet,
deep breathing and exercise are
always outside the conventional treatment armamentarium.
Alternative medicine can be researched enough
to be incorporated into the mainstream."
- Ann Fonfa

"We know from testing, using body burden studies,
that there are a LOT of chemicals in our bodies.
Things we clearly don't need to have in our bodies.
We reach a point where too much of these chemicals
will create health problems."
- Ann Fonfa

"We need to move in a positive direction,
eating vegetables, clean air and water,
a small to moderate amount of exercise, detoxification.
Combining that with a mind/body spirit relaxation
is the best approach overall."
- Ann Fonfa

"That's the Lean & Lovely intention -
to change your body by changing the way
you view and treat yourself."
- Neghar Fonooni

"Whether you think you can or you can't, you're probably right."
- Henry Ford

"Dealing with it is the operative word.
I found myself at seven years not battling it.
Not struggling with it.
Not suffering from it.
Not breaking under the burden of it, but dealing with it."
- Michael J. Fox

"Some people die at 25 and aren't buried until 75."
- Benjamin Franklin

"While we may not be able to control all that happens to us,
we can control what happens inside us."
- Benjamin Franklin

"I don't believe in diets."
- Bethenny Frankel

"Never eat while doing something else,
because you won't get
the satisfaction from your food
and you'll be more likely to overeat."
- Bethenny Frankel

"Your diet is a bank account.
Good food choices are good investments."
- Bethenny Frankel

"Changing my diet - first to vegetarian and then later to vegan
made energy almost a non-issue for me.
I'm never tired until the very end of the day,
and that's very different from how I used to be,
even when I thought I ate pretty healthily."
- Matt Frazier

"I do so little 'consumption'
(of TV, news, social media, blogs)
that I don't spend any energy at all on worrying
or thinking about current events."
- Matt Frazier

"There are many who don't understand
that it's possible to eat a healthy, substantial diet
that includes no animal products whatsoever."
- Matt Frazier

"If a box tries to convince you its contents are healthy,
there's a great chance that they're not."
- Yoni Freedhoff

"You shouldn't wish any days away.
You've got fewer than you think."
- Yoni Freedhoff

"Garbage in garbage out."
- George Fuechsel

"Blueberries, strawberries and blackberries are true super foods.
Naturally sweet and juicy, berries are low in sugar
and high in nutrients - they are
among the best foods you can eat."
- Joel Fuhrman

"Food is really and truly the most effective medicine."
- Joel Fuhrman

"Healthy people eating healthy food
should never need to take an antibiotic."
- Joel Fuhrman

"In the future, it's going to become more and more impossible
for the economy to support how expensive medical care is
and the number of sick people we have.
Why don't we just get our population healthier
so we don't need medical care?"
- Joel Fuhrman

"Seeds and nuts are indispensable for cardiovascular health.
The protective properties of nuts against coronary heart disease
were first recognized in the early 1990s,
and a strong body of literature has followed,
confirming these original findings."
- Joel Fuhrman

"The modern diet is grossly deficient in hundreds of important
plant-derived immunity-building compounds which makes us
highly vulnerable to viruses, infections and disease."
- Joel Fuhrman

"To provide optimal levels of protective micronutrients,
a diet must be vegetable-based, not grain-based."
- Joel Fuhrman

"We're not going to find a magic cure for cancer.
We've got to prevent it."
- Joel Fuhrman

"The elements of water that make it good are a pH that's slightly
alkaline and lots of electrons, because electrons are energy."
- Michael Galitzer

"It is health that is real wealth and not pieces of gold and silver."
- Mahatma Gandhi

"There is nothing that wastes the body like worry,
and one who has any faith in God should be ashamed
to worry about anything whatsoever."
- Mahatma Gandhi

"Let your pain birth your purpose.
Let your mess become your message.
Let this be a stepping-stone and not a stumbling block.
Change."
- Tony A. Gaskins Jr.

"To be content doesn't mean you don't desire more,
it means you're thankful for what you have
and patience for what's to come."
- Tony Gaskins, Jr.

"All chronic and degenerative diseases are caused
by two and only two major problems,
toxicity and deficiency."
- Charlotte Gerson

"For any ill individual as well as for someone
in a state of good health,
drinking fresh-made juices processed from
organically grown fruits and vegetables
frequently through each day is critical to
renewing or maintaining wellness."
- Charlotte Gerson

"Gabriel Feldman, M.D., director of the prostate
and colorectal cancer programs
for the American Cancer Society, admits,
'We don't need years of research.
If people would implement what we know today,
cancer rates would drop. It's that simple'.
Dr. Max Gerson was correct in his medical/nutritional
literary presentation of 1958
before the advent of fast food restaurants
and supermarket convenience foods,
and his intuitions are even more accurate today."
- Charlotte Gerson

"Is there a 'vital force' taken into the body from juice drinking?
It's strictly our opinion, but we say 'Yes!'
The live enzymes in vegetables and fruits may be
absorbed into the physical, mental, and spiritual self
and probably do invigorate one's soul."
- Charlotte Gerson

"It's safer to use foods in the most natural form,
combined and mixed by nature and raised,
if possible, by an organic gardening process,
thus obeying the laws of nature."
- Charlotte Gerson

"It's the doctor's duty to activate and reactivate
the body's own healing mechanism."
- Charlotte Gerson

"No attempt should be made to cure the body
without curing the soul',
wrote Plato nearly 2,400 years ago.
Body and mind are inseparable;
they sicken together and must be healed together."
- Charlotte Gerson

"When you change your diet,
you can change your entire physiology and you can heal."
- Charlotte Gerson

"You can't keep one disease and heal two others.
When the body heals, it heals everything."
- Charlotte Gerson

"You can't trash and pollute your body
and expect to have perfect health."
- Charlotte Gerson

"Stay close to nature and her eternal laws will protect you."
- Max Gerson

"Whoever will correct his diet to a reasonable extent,
take reasonable exercise, and keep his digestive tract
absolutely clean, need have no fear of cancer."
- Max Gerson

"Faith is a knowledge within the heart, beyond the reach of proof."
- Khalil Gibran

"Ask for help.
The power of teamwork is staggering and rewarding."
- DonnaLyn Giegerich

"Kick Cancer Overboard and celebrate life!"
- DonnaLyn Giegerich

"Never underestimate your ability to help someone else
during and after your challenge. Self healing in action."
- DonnaLyn Giegerich

"Medical miracles are happening
in talent and technology daily.
Chose to live in hope to cope
and then fiercely advocate for yourself."
- DonnaLyn Giegerich

"Selfcare is the new healthcare.
Yoga helped save our lives!"
- DonnaLyn Giegerich

"97 percent of the time chemotherapy does not work.
So why is it still used?
There's one reason and one reason only...money."
- Peter Glidden

"Chronic illness is not caused by a bad gene,
or a Gypsy curse, nor is it a function of aging.
Chronic disease is caused by chronic nutrient deficiencies."
- Peter Glidden

"Elegantly simple in its philosophy,
Dr. Wallach's Medical Nutrition Method
professes the following:
The human body requires 91
essential nutrients to function properly.
It is impossible to get all 91 of
these nutrients from our food.
With the passage of time,
unless nutritional supplements are added into the diet,
the body will develop nutrient deficiencies.
When the nutrient deficiencies get big enough,
something breaks, and disease is borne.
If the deficient nutrients are put back into the body before
the diseased tissue reaches its point of no return,
the body will repair itself and eliminate the disease."
- Peter Glidden

"Proper nutrition is the KEY to health and longevity.
It is the magic bullet that eliminates most chronic disease
as most chronic disease is caused by nutrient deficiencies."
- Peter Glidden

"The only way to have a truly integrated medical model in this
country is for ALL medical disciplines to have
equal protection under the law,
equal rates of insurance coverage,
and equal amounts of research dollars, more or less.
Then the marketplace would naturally sort itself out."
- Peter Glidden

"Almost as soon as I went vegan,
people started telling me that my skin looked great,
and that I appeared younger, slimmer, and healthier.
I'm convinced that of all the changes I've made to my lifestyle,
it's the adoption of a vegan diet that has been best for me
- physically, mentally, and certainly spiritually."
- Stephen Glover (aka Steve-O)

"It is difficult to say what is impossible, for the dream of yesterday
is the hope of today and the reality of tomorrow."
- Robert H. Goddard

"Cancer care will advance patient by patient.
As each cancer patient recovers his or her health,
thanks to alternative medicine, and tells a friend and
the family doctor, this will transform Western medicine."
- Burton Goldberg

"Doctors don't want to rock the boat.
They don't want to risk that the FDA will punish them
or their state medical board will yank away their license.
And I don't blame them."
- Burton Goldberg

"Have you ever had a conventional doctor
urge you to eat organic food?"
- Burton Goldberg

"Nothing helps the liver clean out faster, more efficiently,
and more effectively, than coffee enemas."
- Nicholas Gonzalez

"I did this book 'Harvest for Hope,'
and I learned so much about food.
And one thing I learned is that we have the guts
not of a carnivore, but of an herbivore.
Herbivore guts are very long because they have
to get the last bit of nutrition out of leaves and things."
- Jane Goodall

"If you have health, you truly have everything."
- Janice Gordon

"Age is a question of mind over matter.
If you don't mind, it doesn't matter."
- Jon Gordon

"A smooth ocean never made a skilled surfer
and a struggle-free existence
never made a meaningful, great life."
- Jon Gordon

"Decide right now the age you want to be."
- Jon Gordon

"Forgiveness is for yourself, not for them."
- Jon Gordon

"I have found that
the more often I live in the 'now',
the more energy I have.
Energy spent in the past or future is worthless now.
It's like investing money in a company
that already went bankrupt
or hasn't even been created yet."
- Jon Gordon

"It takes a lot more energy to keep positive energy
out of our lives than it does to let it in."
- Jon Gordon

"The energy we project is the energy we receive.
We are like a movie projector and what we project on
to the world's movie screen is what the world sees."
- Jon Gordon

"I want to focus my whole life first of all,
to understand cancer better
and what would be the best form of therapy.
Because a lot of patients,
they are very afraid of cancer."
- Robert Gorter

"Often in medical school it is portrayed
that fever is the cause of illness,
but it's the opposite."
- Robert Gorter

"You stop moving, you're dead.
Then you're no fun."
- Brogan Graham

"As a retired physician, I can honestly say
that unless you are in a serious accident,
your best chance of living to a ripe old age is to
avoid doctors and hospitals and learn nutrition,
herbal medicine and other forms of natural medicine
unless you are fortunate enough to
have a naturopathic physician available.
Almost all drugs are toxic and are designed
only to treat symptoms and not to cure anyone."
- Allan Greenberg

"Exercise is non negotiable,
an appointment you will not miss."
- Bob Greene

"My own prescription for health is less paperwork
and more running barefoot through the grass."
- Leslie Grimutter

"One must not forget that recovery is brought about
not by the physician, but by the sick man himself.
He heals himself, by his own power,
exactly as he walks by means of his own power,
or eats, or thinks, breathes or sleeps."
- Georg Groddeck

"By cleansing your body on a regular basis and eliminating
as many toxins as possible from your environment,
your body can begin to heal itself, prevent disease,
and become stronger and more resilient
than you ever dreamed possible!"
- Edward Group III

"No disease can exist inside of a clean body."
- Edward F. Group III

"What we found with evaluating over 100,000 liver cleanses is
liver cleansing is probably one of the most effective ways of
boosting your self-healing mechanism.
Each liver cleanse is going to boost the liver production
and efficiency by 10 to 15 percent,
which means another thing we found in research
is that most cancer and degenerative disease patients
need multiple liver cleanses."
- Edward F. Group III

"We are all living in a toxic world,
the world is sick, the world has cancer now,
the soil is sick, the air is contaminated,
all we can do is keep our bodies clean
and our self healing mechanism strong...
no disease can exist in a clean body."
- Edward F. Group III

"Hate less, live longer."
- Terri Guillemets

"Health is a relationship between you and your body."
- Terri Guillemets

"Our bodies run on the fresh green fuel of the land."
- Terri Guillemets

"When it comes to eating right and exercising,
there is no 'I'll start tomorrow'.
Tomorrow is disease."
- Terri Guillemets

"Life can pull you down,
but running always lifts you up."
- Jenny Hadfield

"Living in the moment could be the meaning of life."
- Jenny Hadfield

"Music is therapy. Music moves people.
It connects people in ways that no other medium can.
It pulls heart strings. It acts as medicine."
- Ben William Haggerty (aka Macklemore)

"America's health care system is in crisis
precisely because we systematically
neglect wellness and prevention."
- Tom Harkin

"If we are serious about combating the childhood
obesity epidemic and improving child nutrition,
then everyone must chip in -
parents, schools, and yes even Congress."
- Tom Harkin

"Let's face it, in America today
we don't have a health care system,
we have a sick care system."
- Tom Harkin

"Parents should know that our schools
are now one of the largest sources of
unhealthy food for their kids."
- Tom Harkin

"This study shows that when it comes to diet and obesity,
American parents are woefully uninformed."
- Tom Harkin

"Would anyone advocate that we take the fences
off the playground for elementary schools
and just let kids run around in the streets?...
By the same token, why would we allow schools
to sort of poison our kids with junk food?"
- Tom Harkin

"For me, working out is a form of therapy.
It's cathartic for me; it's a good stress reliever.
I know that when I go to the gym I am taking care of myself,
and I know I'll feel so much better afterwards."
- Bob Harper

"I believe in the power of the human spirit."
- Bob Harper

"You can't be a parent and say,
'I need you to be more active and I need you to eat right,'
when you're still choosing to have poor eating habits."
- Bob Harper

"Don't miss your life."
- Valerie Harper

"Hope is important."
- Jackie Hekneby

"I would say think outside the box.
A lot people don't dare because they
really were brought up in our society
to respect our parents and our teachers
and the police and then the doctors,
and people are not used to thinking for themselves.
But you need to think for yourself and do your own research."
- Jackie Hekneby

"The best research is in Ty's book <u>Step Outside the Box</u>.
That is all done for us.
I would say just go organic food,
organic products for hair and skin products.
And boost your immune system with the best possible
plant in the world: moringa oleifera, I would recommend.
And detoxification is also done naturally by moringa oleifera.
Drink only purified water, and exercise or go for gentle walks..."
- Jackie Hekneby

"Strength is born in the deep silence
of long-suffering hearts; not amidst joy."
- Felicia Hemans

"Being in control of your life
and having realistic expectations
about your day-to-day challenges are
the keys to stress management,
which is perhaps the most important ingredient
to living a happy, healthy and rewarding life."
- Marilu Henner

"Foods high in bad fats, sugar and chemicals are
directly linked to many negative emotions,
whereas whole, natural foods rich in nutrients -
foods such as fruits, vegetables, grains and legumes
contribute to greater energy and positive emotions."
- Marilu Henner

"Often when a person can't get past stress,
she will turn to overeating, drinking or smoking,
which can become a greater problem
than the stress itself."
- Marilu Henner

"The biggest reason most people fail is that
they try to fix too much at once
- join a gym, get out of debt,
floss after meals and have thinner thighs in 30 days."
- Marilu Henner

"When health is absent, wisdom cannot reveal itself,
art cannot manifest, strength cannot fight,
wealth becomes useless,
and intelligence cannot be applied."
- Herophilus

"Any disease starts with cellular imbalances
years in advance."
- Raymond Hilu

"A wise man should consider that health
is the greatest of human blessings,
and learn how by his own thought
to derive benefit from his illnesses."
- Hippocrates

"If we could give every individual the right amount
of nourishment and exercise,
not too little and not too much,
we would have found the safest way to health."
- Hippocrates

"Natural forces within us are
the true healers of disease."
- Hippocrates

"Walking is man's best medicine."
- Hippocrates

"Whenever a doctor cannot do good,
he must be kept from doing harm."
- Hippocrates

"It's not all about the scale.
It's about what you're made of!"
- Cassey Ho

"Don't strive for perfection. It doesn't exist.
Strive for a better you. That's always in reach."
- Brett Hoebel

"Food is a lot of people's therapy -
when we say comfort food, we really mean that.
It's releasing dopamine and serotonin
in your brain that makes you feel good."
- Brett Hoebel

"If you think of exercise as a 60-minute commitment
3 times a week at the gym,
you're missing the point completely.
If you think that going on a diet
has something to do with nutrition,
you don't see the forest through the trees.
It is a lifestyle. I know it sounds cliche,
but you have to find things you love to do."
- Brett Hoebel

"If I could give one tip for people -
it's not an exercise or nutrition regimen.
It's to walk your talk and believe in yourself,
because at the end of the day,
the dumbbell and diet don't get you in shape.
It's your accountability to your word."
- Brett Hoebel

"If you don't have an emotional connection
to why you are trying to accomplish your goals,
the odds are you won't reach them or will quit trying."
- Brett Hoebel

"You need to put what you learn into practice
and do it over and over again until it's a habit.
I always say, 'Seeing is not believing. Doing is believing.'
There is a lot to learn about fitness,
nutrition and emotions,
but once you do, you can master them
instead of them mastering you."
- Brett Hoebel

"I'm not sure what Essiac does to extend cancer survival,
and for all we know it may not have this effect.
On the other hand, it's not toxic
and my patients have reported
feeling good while taking it,
so why not support them?"
- Abram Hoffer

"Cancer is a journey, but you walk the road alone.
There are many places to stop
along the way and get nourishment
- you just have to be willing to take it."
- Emily Hollenberg

"In our fast-forward culture,
we have lost the art of eating well.
Food is often little more than fuel to pour down the hatch
while doing other stuff - surfing the Web,
driving, walking along the street.
Dining al desko is now the norm in many workplaces.
All of this speed takes a toll.
Obesity, eating disorders and poor nutrition are rife."
- Carl Honore

"The bloodstream is known as the 'river of life',
and it is the purity of this river which determines,
almost entirely, the health -
mental and physical of the individual."
- Ross Horne

"The brain is a giant immune system gland that
operates on hope, joy, and optimism.
The gland turns off in response to mental attitudes
of fear and depression.
The question is raised as to how many people are dying
because they have been programmed to die.
The observation is made that doctors who tell their patients
they have a terminal disease are programming their patients to die."
- Ross Horne

"Don't just kind of do it!"
- Tony Horton

"Do your best and forget the rest."
- Tony Horton

"A combination of laetrile, Gerson, enzymes and
Coley type vaccines would cure over 95% of cancers."
- Frank Hourigan

"All the great agricultural systems which have survived
have made it their business never to deplete the earth of its fertility
without at the same time beginning the process of restoration."
- Albert Howard

"Artificial manures lead inevitably to artificial nutrition, artificial food,
artificial animals and finally to artificial men and women."
- Albert Howard

"The most important possession of a country is its population.
If this is maintained in health and vigor everything else will follow;
if this is allowed to decline nothing, not even great riches,
can save the country from eventual ruin."
- Albert Howard

"Tell a victim he is hopeless and the will to live becomes paralyzed.
Show him a way out, strip him of fear and hysteria,
give him even a forlorn hope, and the will to live is stimulated.
It becomes a powerful ally in the battle against death."
- Harry A. Hoxsey

"Have you ever thought why
the cancer epidemic is on the rise?
In spite of all efforts to eradicate it?"
- Jenny Hrbacek

"If you have health, you probably will be happy,
and if you have health and happiness,
you have the wealth you need,
even if it is not all you want."
- Elbert Hubbard

"The health care system is really designed to
reward you for being unhealthy. If you are a healthy person
and work hard to be healthy, there are no benefits."
- Mike Huckabee

"We don't have a health care crisis, we have a health crisis!"
- Mike Huckabee

"Oh, my friend,
it's not what they take away from you that counts
- it's what you do with what you have left."
- Hubert Humphrey

"The greatest healing therapy is friendship and love."
- Hubert Humphrey

"The groundwork of all happiness is health."
- Leigh Hunt

"Children with obesity and diabetes live harder poorer lives,
they often don't finish school and earn much less
than their healthy counterparts."
- Mark Hyman

"I don't need the fillers, additives, excessive amounts of sugars,
fats, salts and other measures taken to taint
the natural goodness of real food."
- Mark Hyman

"It seems that for many the cure to acne
is at the end of their fork,
not in a prescription pad."
- Mark Hyman

"Lifestyle change and changes in diet work faster,
better and more cheaply than any medication
and are as effective or more effective than gastric bypass
without any side effects or long-term complications."
- Mark Hyman

"My advice is to give up stevia, aspartame, sucralose,
sugar alcohols like xylitol and malitol,
and all of the other heavily-used
and marketed sweeteners unless you want
to slow down your metabolism,
gain weight, and become an addict."
- Mark Hyman

"Paradoxically Americans are becoming both more obese
and more nutrient deficient at the same time.
Obese children eating processed foods are nutrient depleted
and increasingly get scurvy and rickets,
diseases we thought were left behind
in the 19th and 20th centuries."
- Mark Hyman

"Part of my training was learning how to refer patients to
cardiologists for heart problems, gastroenterologists
for stomach issues, and rheumatologists for joint pain.
Given that most physicians were trained this way,
it's no wonder that the average Medicare patient has
six doctors and is on five different medications."
- Mark Hyman

"Placing too much emphasis on a yes/no diagnosis,
meaning you either have a disease or you don't,
can lead even the most well-meaning physicians to miss
underlying causes and early warning signs of illness."
- Mark Hyman

"Seems you can't outsmart Mother Nature."
- Mark Hyman

"Stay away from milk. It is nature's perfect food
- but only if you are a calf."
- Mark Hyman

"The best advice is to avoid foods
with health claims on the label,
or better yet avoid foods
with labels in the first place."
- Mark Hyman

"The body maintains balance
in only a handful of ways.
At the end of the day, disease occurs when
these basic systems are out of whack."
- Mark Hyman

"The food industry profits from providing
poor quality foods with poor nutritional value
that people eat a lot of."
- Mark Hyman

"The very fact that we are having a national conversation
about what we should eat, that we are struggling
with the question about what the best diet is,
is symptomatic of how far we have strayed
from the natural conditions that gave rise to our species,
from the simple act of eating real, whole, fresh food."
- Mark Hyman

"The way most doctors practice
medicine right now isn't working."
- Mark Hyman

"When it becomes a revolutionary act to eat real food,
we are in trouble."
- Mark Hyman

"You can't exercise your way out of a bad diet."
- Mark Hyman

"The good-news stories in medicine are
early detection, early intervention."
- Thomas R. Insel

"Health is a state of complete harmony
of the body, mind and spirit.
When one is free from physical disabilities
and mental distractions, the gates of the soul open."
- B. K. Iyengar

"Burning fat is simple and straightforward if you eat the foods
we were built to eat and get off the couch every once in a while.
There is hope."
- Abel James

"Grains rapidly elevate your blood sugar and cause
your body to store fat, rather than burn it.
How do you fatten a cow? Feed it grains.
How do you fatten a human? Feed it grains."
- Abel James

"If you can't pronounce an ingredient (or five) on the label,
you probably shouldn't eat it."
- Abel James

"In the United States, Big Food doesn't even have to tell you
which foods contain this genetically altered corn on the label or
whether it was used to feed the animals you're eating.
No wonder Europe won't import our food.
Even China, the country known for feeding poultry
feces to its farmed fish, banned our meat
and much of our processed food.
We can do better."
- Abel James

"It's important to note the few staples of the Standard American Diet
- namely corn, wheat, and soy are not produced in such
massive quantities because they're healthy.
They're produced because they make money for rich people."
- Abel James

"Modern food manufacturers have overwhelmed grocery store
shelves with foods that are nutrient poor,
rotten, spoiled, dead, old, and contaminated
with antibiotics, chemicals, and growth hormones.
Refining has also brought us spectacularly cheap, pervasive,
and fattening ingredients: namely white flour, white sugar,
high fructose corn syrup, and industrial seed oils."
- Abel James

"One hundred years from now, medical doctors,
scientists, nutritionists, and the general public
will be puzzled and astounded by how few of us were
able to grasp the obvious: high-carb, low-fat diets
simply do not work long-term."
- Abel James

"Leave all the afternoon for exercise and recreation,
which are as necessary as reading.
I will rather say more necessary
because health is worth more than learning."
- Thomas Jefferson

"The doctor of the future will give no medicine,
but will interest his patients
in the care of the human frame,
in diet, and in the cause
and prevention of disease."
- Thomas Jefferson

"Walking is the best possible exercise.
Habituate yourself to walk very far."
- Thomas Jefferson

"We never repent of having eaten too little."
- Thomas Jefferson

"Choose quality fuel: All calories are not equal.
1,500 calories of processed food has a completely
different effect on your body than 1,500 calories of fresh
fruits and vegetables, lean cuts of meat and whole grains.
The fiber and most of the nutrients are removed from most
processed foods like snack bars, crackers, bagels, chips,
bread, muffins and cereal, so when you eat these foods
your body recognizes them as sugar, spiking your insulin
and causing you to crave more food."
- Jeanette Jenkins

"Eat until you're satisfied and stop before you're full.
The stomach is made of smooth muscle,
and when you overeat you stretch the smooth muscle
of your stomach, which in turn increases your appetite.
Always stop eating as soon as you feel satisfied
to avoid stretching your stomach.
You can always eat again in two hours."
- Jeanette Jenkins

"Every living cell in your body is made from the food you eat.
If you consistently eat junk food
then you'll have a junk body."
- Jeanette Jenkins

"When you choose to perceive a situation in life,
you then have to live in that perception,
so if you choose to look for the negative,
then you will live in a negative experience,
and if you choose to look for the positive,
then you will live in a positive experience.
The choice is yours, so choose wisely."
- Jeanette Jenkins

"A negative thought can kill you
faster than a bad germ."
- Antonio Jimenez

"When a person goes into the operating room,
he will realize that there is one book
that he has yet to finish reading
- 'Book of Healthy Life'."
- Steve Jobs

"When we take the sugar out, we are taking away
the preferred fuel source for the cancer cells."
- David C. Jockers

"Music has healing power.
It has the ability to take people
out of themselves for a few hours."
- Elton John

"Family, nature and health all go together."
- Olivia Newton John

"I always suggest that when you're going through cancer
to find something in your day that makes you feel centered
and that makes you feel good."
- Olivia Newton John

"I live every day to its fullest extent
and I don't sweat the small stuff."
- Olivia Newton John

"I love life and nothing intimidates me anymore."
- Olivia Newton John

"I made an album of healing music called
'Grace and Gratitude' that came from my soul."
- Olivia Newton John

"I've always been aware of my health -
when you are having to go on stage and perform,
you need to be feeling good -
but when I was diagnosed with a
life-threatening illness,
I became really, really conscious of my health."
- Olivia Newton John

"My cancer scare changed my life.
I'm grateful for every new, healthy day I have.
It has helped me prioritize my life."
- Olivia Newton John

"My family and friends were definitely the key to my recovery.
One thing that I do suggest is that anyone dealing with a
life-threatening illness like cancer
choose a point person for people to call
to find out how you are doing -
a sister, brother, mother, father,
daughter, son, or close friend."
- Olivia Newton John

"Hope is not the conviction that something will turn out well,
but the certainty that something makes sense
regardless of how it turns out."
- Barbara Johnson

"Mammograms actually cause cancer."
- Ben Johnson

"All movement creates momentum.
All momentum is progress."
- Chalene Johnson

"Positive energy is your priceless life force. Protect it.
Don't allow people to draw from your reserves;
select friends who recharge your energies...
I'm not asking you to cut people out of your life,
but I am asking you to invest your time with people
who will push you to be your best.
Winners love to see other people win."
- Chalene Johnson

"The right habits are the only things that
separate you from the life you want to live."
- Chalene Johnson

"The American College of Sports Medicine found that
the productivity of people after exercise was an average
of 65 percent higher than those who did not exercise.
If I have something that's really bothering me,
so much that it almost hurts my head to try to sort it out,
I always find the solution in a puddle of sweat!
Intense exercise is like taking a magic pill that
gives you the ability to solve problems like a superhero."
- Chalene Johnson

"The vital difference between dreamers and achievers
boils down to some very basic, simple habits.
People with clear, 'written-out' goals who consistently honor
their defined priorities tend to get results faster than others,
and enjoy a greater level of happiness and long-term
success in all areas of life.
Yet most of us have never been formally taught
a system of goal-setting and mastery that
can be applied to health and fitness."
- Chalene Johnson

"Your health and fitness do not exist independently
of the other areas of your life."
- Chalene Johnson

"I make sure I get a lot of vegetables, a lot of fruit.
I am a big fruit man; I am a vegetable man, anyway."
- Earvin "Magic" Johnson Jr.

"The human body has been designed to resist
an infinite number of changes and attacks
brought about by its environment.
The secret of good health lies
in successful adjustment to
changing stresses on the body."
- Harry J. Johnson

"If fear is cultivated it will become stronger,
if faith is cultivated it will achieve mastery."
- John Paul Jones

"The one thing I learned from this trip is that
there is not one cure for cancer,
there are a billion cures for cancer."
- Travis Jones

"Your body hears everything your mind says."
- Naomi Judd

"I speak as a cancer patient who 7 years ago
was sent home to die by a doctor who told me
there was nothing more traditional medicine could do for me...
One of the doctors who performed my surgery told me
that I had the fastest growing type known to man
and cobalt and chemo would not help me...
If I had accepted the advice of my doctor,
if I had not been directed to Dr. Kelley,
I would be another cancer statistic."
- Pat Judson

"Altogether, our modern inclination toward sloth,
the easy availability of processed food,
and the prevalence of life-saving medical treatments
have made us a long-lived, unhealthy people."
- Scott Jurek

"She died on March 22. Those last hours I didn't stop stroking her
hair or telling her, 'Don't worry, I'm here'. I told her that I was a good
cook because of her. I told her I ate fresh fruit and vegetables
because of her. I told her I ran because of her. I told her I could still
picture the little garden on our dead-end road. I could feel the rough
wooden spoon, my hands clutching it, hers covering mine. I told her
I remembered that, how warm her hands felt. I told her I loved her
and that she would always be with me. I didn't tell her I was lost."
- Scott Jurek

"We can live as we were meant to live
- simply, joyously, of and on the earth.
We can live with all our effort and with pure happiness."
- Scott Jurek

"You never know how strong you are
until being strong is the only choice you have."
- Scott Jurek

"Toughness is in the soul and spirit, not in muscles."
- Alex Karras

"When written in Chinese, the word 'crisis'
is composed of two characters -
one represents danger, the other represents opportunity."
- John F. Kennedy

"Make a list of what is really important to you. Embody it."
- Jon Kabat-Zinn

"Symptoms of illness and distress,
plus your feelings about them,
can be viewed as messengers coming to tell you
something important about your body or about your mind.
In the old days, if a king didn't like the message he was given,
he would sometimes have the messenger killed.
This is tantamount to suppressing your symptoms
or your feelings because they are unwanted.
Killing the messenger and denying the message
or raging against it are not intelligent ways
of approaching healing."
- Jon Kabat-Zinn

"We take care of the future best
by taking care of the present now."
- Jon Kabat-Zinn

"I can't provide you with the motivation to want to make
changes in your life - that has to come from within you.
YOU have to decide that exercising
and eating healthy will be a priority in your life."
- Steve Kamb

"Don't give in to just a treatment that's promised."
- Pamela Kelsey

"What we have in the United States is not so much a
health-care system as a disease-care system."
- Edward Kennedy

"Physical fitness is not only one of the most
important keys to a healthy body,
it is the basis of dynamic and
creative intellectual activity."
- John F. Kennedy

"I try my best to eat healthy the majority of the time
so that I feel good and have more energy.
I am so passionate about eating healthily,
I am actually certified in nutrition.
I try my best to eat organic whenever possible,
but it's important not to be too strict about it.
Just do the best you can."
- Miranda Kerr

"I've always had a burning desire to help people
and make a difference in the world.
I didn't know how I could do that in modeling
when it can be such a fake world.
But my dad told me I could make a difference
by being true to myself and teaching people
what I've learnt about spirituality, health and nutrition."
- Miranda Kerr

"Problems either have solutions - or they don't.
Either you can do something about them
here and now - or you can't.
If you can do something here and now about them,
then do it - even if it's just a first step.
It saps your energy to be worried or anxious about a problem.
Do what you can do, but don't be addicted to the results
or you will create more worry for yourself."
- Ken Keyes

"The worst thing in your life may contain the seeds of the best."
- Joe Kogel

"There have been some good studies done in California with
Hispanic parents where in the course of a year,
they have changed their entire nutritional intake for the better.
The kid becomes, in a sense, the bridge
between the educational process and the home."
- C. Everett Koop

"Drinking freshly made juices and eating enough
whole foods to provide adequate fiber is a
sensible approach to a healthful diet."
- Jay Kordich

"Juicing is the key to a long, healthy, disease-free life."
- Jay Kordich

"If everyone on a standard American diet stopped eating cereal
grains, industrial seed oils, and excess sugar tomorrow,
I'm willing to bet that the rates of obesity, diabetes, heart disease,
and just about every chronic inflammatory disease
would plummet over the next decade."
- Chris Kresser

"Over the last several years I've come to believe that
chronic stress and the cascade of changes it causes in the body
is second only to diet as the primary cause of modern disease."
- Chris Kresser

"There is strong evidence to support the influence of
our food choices on the health and vibrancy of our skin."
- Chris Kresser

"A balanced life is like a three legged stool. Each leg - nutrition,
fitness and wellness is necessary and supports the other."
- Ellie Krieger

"In my food world, there is no fear or guilt,
only joy and balance.
So no ingredient is ever off-limits.
Rather, all of the recipes here follow my
Usually-Sometimes-Rarely philosophy.
Notice there is no Never."
- Ellie Krieger

"I run 30 minutes in the morning,
and I'm literally the slowest person out there.
For example, just today, old people
were speed-walking past me, and I was like,
'This is pathetic,' but then I thought,
'I'm out here, I'm moving my body and I get to be outside'."
- Ellie Krieger

"I think that learning about nutrition transformed
my relationship with food in a healthy way."
- Ellie Krieger

"So often, people's perceptions of healthy food is that
there must be some compromise in taste and enjoyment,
but I try to show that it is all interconnected,
that delicious food can also be healthy food."
- Ellie Krieger

"To get people to eat well,
Don't say a word about health,
Just cook fantastic food for them."
- Ellie Krieger

"It is no measure of health to be well adjusted
to a profoundly sick society."
- J Krishnamurti

"There's more to life than training,
but training is what puts more in your life."
- Brooks Kubik

"I do it as a therapy. I do it as something to keep me alive.
We all need a little discipline.
Exercise is my discipline."
- Jack LaLanne

"Look at the average American diet:
ice cream, butter, cheese, whole milk, all this fat.
People don't realize how much of this stuff you
get by the end of the day.
High blood pressure is from all this high-fat eating."
- Jack LaLanne

"Probably millions of Americans got up this morning
with a cup of coffee, a cigarette and a donut.
No wonder they are sick and fouled up."
- Jack LaLanne

"Yes, exercise is the catalyst.
That's what makes everything happen:
your digestion, your elimination,
your sex life, your skin, hair,
everything about you depends on circulation.
And how do you increase circulation?"
- Jack LaLanne

"No one has ever drowned in his own sweat."
- Ann Landers

"I run six-to-eight miles a day,
plus weights and aerobics in the lunch hour."
- Hugh Laurie

"When we are properly educated,
the scale weight can actually be an
incredibly valuable tool to gauge health and fitness progress.
Frequent self-monitoring can improve
self-awareness by alerting the individual to
subtle weight increases that can then be
nipped in the bud via dietary and exercise intervention."
- Sohee Lee

"Now there are more overweight people
in America than average-weight people.
So overweight people are now average.
Which means you've met your New Year's resolution."
- Jay Leno

"If you don't have confidence, you'll always find a way not to win."
- Carl Lewis

"I've found that a person does not need protein from meat
to be a successful athlete. In fact, my best year of
track competition was the first year I ate a vegan diet.
- Carl Lewis

"And in the end, it's not the years in your life that count.
It's the life in your years."
- Abraham Lincoln

"I workout for what it does to my mind.
My physique is just a bi-product of
all of my hard work in the gym."
- Tom Link

"When you switch the lens and heal your mind of negativity,
it actually helps heal your body of exhaustion, aches, and pains."
- Frank Lipman

"To insure good health:
eat lightly, breathe deeply, live moderately,
cultivate cheerfulness, and maintain an interest in life."
- William Londen

"We are the authors of our own lives; it falls only to us."
- Rob Lowe

"I'm a vegetarian, and I long for people to eat less meat,
but the thing to do is not to go, 'Eat! Less! Meat!' It's to say,
'I am fit as a flea and I'm 63, I haven't eaten meat for 40 years,
and I never get diseases, I'm never ill, and I'm full of energy.
So how's about that?"
- Joanna Lumley

"The greatest miracle on Earth is the human body.
It is stronger and wiser than you may realize,
and improving its ability to self heal is within your control."
- Fabrizio Mancini

"Fear can only grow in darkness.
Once you face fear with light, you win."
- Steve Maraboli

"Forget yesterday - it has already forgotten you.
Don't sweat tomorrow - you haven't even met.
Instead, open your eyes and your heart
to a truly precious gift - today."
- Steve Maraboli

"God's word is not just to be heard and repeated,
it is to be breathed, lived, and emulated with each action."
- Steve Maraboli

"Incredible change happens in your life when you decide
to take control of what you do have power over
instead of craving control over what you don't."
- Steve Marabol

"I promise you nothing is as chaotic as it seems.
Nothing is worth your health. Nothing is worth
poisoning yourself into stress, anxiety, and fear."
- Steve Marabodi

"Just an observation:
it is impossible to be both grateful and depressed.
Those with a grateful mindset tend
to see the message in the mess.
And even though life may knock them down,
the grateful find reasons,
if even small ones, to get up."
- Steve Maraboli

"Learn from the past,
but don't live in the past."
- Steve Maraboli

"Let today be the day you stop being haunted
by the ghost of yesterday.
Holding a grudge & harboring anger/resentment
is poison to the soul.
Get even with people...
but not those who have hurt us,
forget them, instead get even with
those who have helped us."
- Steve Maraboli

"Life doesn't get easier or more forgiving,
we get stronger and more resilient."
- Steve Maraboli

"Sometimes life knocks you on your ass...
get up, get up, get up!!!
Happiness is not the absence of problems,
it's the ability to deal with them."
- Steve Maraboli

"The purpose of fear is to raise your awareness
not to stop your progress."
- Steve Maraboli

"We can't undo a single thing we have ever done,
but we can make decisions today that propel us
to the life we want and towards the healing we need."
- Steve Maraboli

"When a new day begins,
dare to smile gratefully."
- Steve Marabol

"When you arise in the morning,
think of what a precious privilege it is to be alive
- to breathe, to think, to enjoy, to love
- then make that day count!"
- Steve Maraboli

"You are beautiful. Your beauty,
just like your capacity for life, happiness,
and success, is immeasurable."
- Steve Maraboli

"You have been blessed with immeasurable power
to make positive changes in your life."
- Steve Maraboli

"You have the ability to choose your reactions."
- Steve Maraboli

"You must learn to let go. Release the stress.
You were never in control anyway."
- Steve Maraboli

"Your fear is 100% dependent
on you for its survival."
- Steve Maraboli

"There is no medicine like hope,
no incentive so great,
and no tonic so powerful as
expectation of something tomorrow."
- Orison Swett Marden

"The greatest wealth is health."
- Publius Vergilius Maro (aka Virgil)

"The keys to patience are acceptance and faith.
Accept things as they are, and look
realistically at the world around you.
Have faith in yourself and
in the direction you have chosen."
- Ralph Marston

"I'd love to open up sessions at a Boys and Girls Club
or something where kids can learn nutrition
and how to exercise in a fun way.
Especially for young guys.
I'd love to be an inspiration."
- James Maslow

"The aim of medicine is to prevent
disease and prolong life,
the ideal of medicine is to
eliminate the need of a physician."
- William J. Mayo

"Cook what's fresh for the day.
When you're using fresh fruits, vegetables, and foods,
it's easier to keep the weight off.
And I eat whatever I want - just not a ton of it."
- Debi Mazar

"I gave up all the beer. I gave up the wine.
I haven't drank for six months, more.
I gave up coffee. I gave up all sugary products.
I gave up all processed foods, processed meats.
And now I've just got a very basic diet of
vegetables, fruit, my vitamins and minerals.
And I might have meat now once a week, organic meats,
since I got my results on the 8th of May.
And I have fish maybe once or twice a week
since I got the results. But I have no grains.
- Henry McElligot

"I just look at this experience of the last
six months as a wake-up call.
It's just a wake-up call.
It's just another chapter in my life,
and I take it as a challenge.
Through the last six months,
I had to be mentally very strong.
And that has helped me - being mentally strong."
- Henry McElligot

"I refuse the chemo treatment and radiation.
I'm going to do some research myself and seek
a natural alternative to the chemo and the radiation."
- Henry McElligot

"I was diagnosed to die in a few months.
I'm fully healthy. I'm leading an active life.
I'm helping hundreds of people. Through information I learned,
I'm teaching hundreds of people and helping them with
their cancer cures through the information I got from Ty's show."
- Henry McElligot

"All the money in the world can't
buy you back good health."
- Reba McEntire

"Where your mind goes...your life goes.
Chart the course for your future by the thoughts
you think about in your mind.
Get in agreement with God and think positive
because when you do,
amazing things will happen in your life
and the lives of those around you!"
- Laura Thompson McFaden

"If we went back to the basics
of vegetables, legumes, grains
- the things closer to the earth,
it's a lot better for the earth and for other people.
We can feed more people,
we can feed the starving people."
- Nellie McKay

"I've never dieted in my life; I like food too much.
I'm just thoughtful about what I eat,
and I'm lucky that I love the taste of vegetables.
I'm certainly not 'actress skinny,' and I never will be.
I'm strong, and my body works great for me."
- Sarah McLachlan

"The only courage that matters is the kind
that gets you from one moment to the next."
- Mignon McLaughlin

"Every day I plant seeds in the Garden of My Dreams!
Cultivating passion and drive to live my Best Self:
Mind, 'Body', & Spirit."
- Ginny Scales Medeiros

"Health and intellect are the two blessings of life."
- Menander

"Eat real food."
- Joseph Mercola

"Heartwarming and inspirational quotes can
always uplift and brighten a person's day!"
- Joseph Mercola

"Making sure you drink enough pure water
is one of the most important and powerful
steps you can take for good health."
- Joseph Mercola

"Read packaged food labels like they're
the hottest thing from Oprah's book club."
- Joseph Mercola

"My model is to help people understand that
they can take control of their health."
- Joseph Mercola

"The typical American gets 95%
of their calories from processed food."
- Joseph Mercola

"Your body was not designed
to sit 8 to 10 hours a day.
It's not just exercise,
its movement that is so critical."
- Joseph Mercola

"Food addiction is VERY real."
- Joseph Mercola

"Having a positive outlook and a cheerful disposition
isn't only a happier way to live your life
- it's a healthier way as well."
- Joseph Mercola

"I'm an advocate for the truth, and the truth is that,
every year, we are spending over $2 trillion in the U.S. alone
for a fatally-flawed health care system that is killing
hundreds of thousands of people every year,
simply because they do not have the understanding,
an awareness, of the alternatives to
potentially-toxic and expensive medications."
- Joseph Mercola

"Mindfulness and meditation are among the
best methods to boost your ability to focus.
Ideally, start your day with a mindfulness 'exercise,'
such as focusing on your breathing for five minutes
before you get out of bed.
This can help you to stay better focused
for the rest of your day."
- Joseph Mercola

"The connection between optimism and
other positive emotions and good health
has been firmly established by
scientific research, and the link appears to
be particularly strong when it comes to
heart health. Being lighthearted, it turns out,
is one of the best ways to protect your heart."
- Joseph Mercola

"A life is either all spiritual or not spiritual at all.
No man can serve two masters.
Your life is shaped by the end you live for.
You are made in the image of what you desire."
- Thomas Merton

"Happiness is not a matter of intensity
but of balance and order and rhythm and harmony."
- Thomas Merton

"Perhaps I am stronger than I think."
- Thomas Merton

"We have what we seek, it is there all the time,
and if we give it time, it will make itself known to us."
- Thomas Merton

"I believe that the greatest gift you can give
your family and the world is a healthy you."
- Joyce Meyer

"It's so important to realize that every time you get upset,
it drains your emotional energy.
Losing your cool makes you tired.
Getting angry a lot messes with your health."
- Joyce Meyer

"There's no happier person than a truly thankful, content person."
- Joyce Meyer

"You cannot have a positive life and a negative mind."
- Joyce Meyer

"I've always believed fitness is an entry point to
help you build that happier, healthier life.
When your health is strong, you're capable of taking risks.
You'll feel more confident to ask for the promotion.
You'll have more energy to be a better mom.
You'll feel more deserving of love."
- Jillian Michaels

"My agenda is trying to help people live a better life."
- Jillian Michaels

"The important thing is not that we can live on hope alone,
but that life is not worth living without it."
- Harvey Milk

"You never know how strong you are
until being strong is the only choice you have."
- Cayla Mills

"Respect your body. Eat well. Dance forever."
- Eliza Gaynor Minden

"Cholesterol does not exist in vegetables.
Vegetables do not clog arteries."
- Jane Velez Mitchell

"The mind has great influence over the body,
and maladies often have their origin there."
- Jean Baptiste Molière

"I love the idea of getting up early on Sundays and
walking to the market to pick up fresh fruits and vegetables.
It's a good way to start my day, and it makes me feel like
I've accomplished something before other people are even awake."
- Mandy Moore

"Every night I watch the nightly news.
It's funded by the pharmaceutical companies.
Virtually every ad is a drug ad.
They get their say every night
on the nightly news through advertising."
- Michael Moore

"If you're in a diabetic or pre-diabetic state,
it's good to have medication to go on for a period of time.
But simply by making the changes - get your sleep,
35 grams of fiber and a half-hour walk
- your cholesterol will come down,
your sugar will come down,
and your blood pressure will come down.
Only the minority of people can't control it."
- Michael Moore

"The number one cause of
bankruptcies is medical bills."
- Michael Moore

"Health messages are simply overwhelmed,
in volume and in effectiveness,
by junk-food ads that often deploy celebrities
or cartoon characters to great effect.
We may know that eating fruits and vegetables is good for us,
but the preponderance of the signals we get
- and especially the signals children get
push us in the direction of junk food."
- Michael Moss

"A study was done which shows the majority of oncologists who
refer patients for chemotherapy for lung cancer would
not themselves take chemotherapy for lung cancer."
- Ralph Moss

"I had a brain cancer specialist
sit in my living room and tell me
he would never take radiation if he had a brain tumor.
And I asked him, 'but, do you send people for radiation?'
and he said, of course.
'I'd be drummed out of the hospital if I didn't."
- Ralph Moss

"Investing in early childhood nutrition
is a surefire strategy.
The returns are incredibly high."
- Anne M. Mulcahy

"Any good health measure,
is an anti-cancer measure."
- Keith Scott Mumby

"If I had to, you know, promote sugar water
or a candy bar in order to race a car,
I wouldn't race a car.
So whenever I hit the race track,
my cars are carrying messages about issues that
I think are important, like renewable energies,
solar power, wind power."
- Leilani Münter

"By eating many fruits and vegetables in place of
fast food and junk food, people could avoid obesity."
- David H. Murdock

"No pills, not even aspirin, and certainly no supplements
ever enter my mouth - everything I need comes from
my fish and vegetarian diet, which incorporates many
different kinds of fruit and vegetables every week."
- David H. Murdock

"Life is too short for long-term grudges."
- Elon Musk

"It is not the calories one should be worried about,
it is the ingredients in our food!"
- Chad Napier

"People want great health!
They want to conquer disease and cancer,
but people do not know or even understand
the importance of Universal Law!"
- Chad Napier

"In order to defeat our greatest enemy of
disease and cancer, we must, first, know our enemy!"
- Chad Napier

"The secret to conquering ANY disease or cancer
is coming to a realization that our entire body
works in unison together.
Treat the body as a whole and a miracle begins to happen!"
- Chad Napier

"Healthy, sustainable food production methods give us food
that is nutritionally better and with fewer pesticides,
antibiotics, and hormones."
- Marion Nestle

"It's time to get the FDA to reverse its 1994 decision
not to label GM foods."
- Marion Nestle

"Going meat-free can make a huge difference.
Studies show that vegetarians are, on average,
10 to 20 pounds lighter than meat-eaters and that
a vegetarian diet reduces our risk of heart disease
by 40 percent and adds seven or more years to our lifespan."
- Ingrid Newkirk

"Real nutrition comes from soybeans, almonds, rice,
and other healthy vegetable sources, not from a cow's udder."
- Ingrid Newkirk

"We are living in a world today where lemonade
is made from artificial flavors and
furniture polish is made from real lemons."
- Alfred Newman

"What does not kill us makes us stronger."
- Friedrich Nietzsche

"As a chemist trained to interpret data,
it is incomprehensible to me
that physicians can ignore the clear evidence that
chemotherapy does much, much more harm than good."
- Alan Nixon

"Growing old is inevitable.
Aging is optional!"
- Christiane Northrup

"If you are constantly around negativity,
that will adversely affect you."
- Christiane Northrup

"Joy is contagious and amplifies
everything else that goes on."
- Christiane Northrup

"People with the most varied social contact
have the best immunity."
- Christiane Northrup

"So much of what we are is about our programming.
What we think about, we focus on;
what we focus on can manifest."
- Christiane Northrup

"The friend who can be silent with us
in a moment of despair or confusion,
who can stay with us in an hour of grief and bereavement,
who can tolerate not knowing... not healing, not curing...
that is a friend who cares."
- Henri Nouwen

"ANY doctor in the United States who cures cancer
using alternative methods will be destroyed.
You cannot name me a doctor doing well with cancer using
alternative therapies that is not under attack.
And I KNOW these people; I've interviewed them."
- Gary Null

"Happiness isn't a state, it's a skill.
It's the skill of knowing how to take what life throws
your way and make the most of it."
- Gary Null

"I can name you sixty doctors treating cancer
with alternative methods. All sixty are under attack.
And yet their patients are alive or improving.
Some have been cured and it's documented."
- Gary Null

"I have a doctor who called me last year.
He listens to the show and personally he lives a healthy life.
And he was angry. And he didn't know what to do. He wanted to
think whether or not he could expose the situation without getting
himself involved. He said, 'I'm giving cancer patients over here at
this major cancer clinic drugs that are killing them, and I can't stop it
because they say the protocol's what's important.'
And I say, 'But the patient's not doing well."
They say, 'The protocol's what's important, not the patient.'
And he said, 'You can't believe what goes on in the name of
medicine and science in this country'."
- Gary Null

"Learn the lesson of your pain."
- Gary Null

"Most fears are just illusions."
- Gary Null

"We went through the records and we found over
five hundred of his patients who were alive and well
five years after their treatment, with no cancer.
And Dr. Burton didn't selectively give us these.
These were 'take what you want.
Here are the patients I treated'.
So there was statistical improvement
- more so than any cancer institution
in the United States could show."
- Gary Null

"All those toxins in your body
are blocking the healing process:
amalgams in your teeth, an infection,
a yeast overgrowth, fluoride, environmental toxins,
pesticides, herbicides, and heavy metals.
They are a road block to your healing."
- Daniel Nuzum

"And let's be clear:
It's not enough just to limit ads
for foods that aren't healthy.
It's also going to be critical
to increase marketing
for foods that are healthy."
- Michelle Obama

"Choose people who lift you up."
- Michelle Obama

"I look at how my kids view exercise.
They have a complete understanding
that nutrition and exercise go hand in hand.
I didn't think like that when I was a kid.
But they have a real consciousness about it
that I'd like to think comes from the years
of attention we've put into this."
- Michelle Obama

"We can make a commitment
to promote vegetables and fruits
and whole grains on every part of every menu.
We can make portion sizes smaller and
emphasize quality over quantity.
And we can help create a culture - imagine this
where our kids ask for healthy options
instead of resisting them."
- Michelle Obama

"When I get up and work out, I'm working out
just as much for my girls as I am for me,
because I want them to see a mother who loves them dearly,
who invests in them, but who also invests in herself.
It's just as much about letting them know
as young women that it is okay to put yourself
a little higher on your priority list."
- Michelle Obama

"Every forkful of what you put in your mouth is either
inflammatory or anti-inflammatory. Make wise choices."
- Tom O'Bryan

"The World Health Organization
tells us the United States ranks
second in overall health care...
second from the bottom."
- Tom O'Bryan

"Health is a unity of mind, body and soul!"
- Kim Oexner

"Without Health there is no Wealth!"
- Kim Oexner

"No pill manufactured can replace the warmth
of the sun and the bounty of nature!"
- Larry Oexner

"Our candle of life lasts just so long.
It is a flicker for some,
a bright shining beacon for others.
The foods we eat,
the physical activity we bestow upon ourselves
and the spiritual message we live by,
makes that candle a bit shorter or a bit longer!"
- Larry Oexner

"Your body is your temple. Your food is your martyr!"
- Larry Oexner

"The public health of five million children
should not be left to luck or chance."
- Jamie Oliver

"Because the biological mechanisms that affect
our health and well-being are so dynamic,
when people change their diet and lifestyle,
they usually feel so much better, so quickly;
it reframes the reason for changing
from fear of dying to joy of living.
Also, the support that patients give
each other is a powerful motivator."
- Dean Ornish

"I grew up in Texas, eating meat five times a day,
and I liked meat. But I began being a vegetarian
when I was 19 because I found that I felt better."
- Dean Ornish

"People who are lonely and depressed are
three to 10 times more likely to get sick and die
prematurely than those who have
a strong sense of love and community.
I don't know any other single factor that affects our health
- for better and for worse to such a strong degree."
- Dean Ornish

"Poor health is not caused by something you don't have;
it's caused by disturbing something that you already have.
Healthy is not something that you need to get,
it's something you have already if you don't disturb it."
- Dean Ornish

"Think about it:
Heart disease and diabetes, which account
for more deaths in the U.S. and worldwide than
teverything else combined, are completely preventable
by making comprehensive lifestyle changes.
Without drugs or surgery."
- Dean Ornish

"It is much more important to know what sort of a patient
has a disease than what sort of a disease a patient has."
- William Osler

"Listen to the patient.
They will tell you what's wrong with them."
- William Osler

"One of the first duties of the physician is to
educate the masses not to take medicine."
- William Osler

"The good physician treats the disease;
the great physician treats
the patient who has the disease."
- William Osler

"A lot of psychological principles
and even medical principles,
you see them coming around to what the Bible
said hundreds of years ago:
a merry heart is good like a medicine."
- Joel Osteen

"Every day is a gift from God.
There's no guarantee of tomorrow, so that tells me
to see the good in this day to make the most of it."
- Joel Osteen

"I think faith is incredibly important because you will become
overwhelmed with what's happening and you will have waves of
grief, but when you turn to your faith, I believe God
will give you waves of grace to get through it."
- Joel Osteen

"Every hour you sit at work
increases your mortality 11 percent.
Think about that."
- Mehmet Oz

"Food is no longer sacred to us:
in becoming too efficient we've changed its nature."
- Mehmet Oz

"If I make your workplace conducive
to walking at lunch,or working out
at some time during the day,
or I get people to use the stairs more
by creating incentives to do such,
then people will start doing it naturally."
- Mehmet Oz

"If you don't know your blood pressure,
it's like not knowing the value of your company."
- Mehmet Oz

"I saw many people who had advanced heart disease
and I was so frustrated because I knew
if they just knew how to do the right thing,
simple lifestyle and diet steps,
that the entire trajectory of their life
and health would have been different."
- Mehmet Oz

"Most allopathic doctors think practitioners
of alternative medicine are all quacks.
They're not. Often they're sharp people
who think differently about disease."
- Mehmet Oz

"People say their weight is genetic.
But it turns out that people who are overweight
don't just have overweight kids.
They also have overweight pets.
That's not genetic."
- Mehmet Oz

"The rule I use is, If it doesn't come out of the ground
looking the way it looks when you eat it, be careful."
- Mehmet Oz

"We are spending most of our time in American health care fixing
the mistakes that either we in the profession are causing or our
patients are, without recognizing it, causing to themselves."
- Mehmet Oz

"We don't need sugar to live,
and we don't need it as a society."
- Mehmet Oz

"Your genetics load the gun. Your lifestyle pulls the trigger."
- Mehmet Oz

"The cases are so frequent in which deep anxiety, deferred hope
and disappointment are quickly followed
by the growth and increase of cancer,
that we can hardly doubt that mental depression
is a weighty additive to the other influences favoring
the development of the cancerous constitution."
- James Paget

"Our body already has this
natural mechanism to fight cancer,
we just have to take care of it."
- Sunil Pai

"With cancer or any other chronic disease,
its all about lowering inflammation
and increasing the immune system response."
- Sunil Pai

"The art of healing comes from nature,
not from the physician.
Therefore the physician must start from nature,
with an open mind."
- Paracelsus

"In faith there is enough light
for those who want to believe and
enough shadows to blind those who don't."
- Blaise Pascal

"You're eating right and exercising regularly.
But there is one barrier in the way to slimming down:
It's our sneaky old nemesis, sugar,
which lies in wait at every turn."
- Harley Pasternak

"To fear is one thing.
To let fear grab you by the tail
and swing you around is another."
- Katherine Paterson

"How you eat determines your mood
and your outlook on life."
- Alexandra Paul

"Sometimes I wake up in the morning & go Ahh...
I don't want to work out!
But I do anyway, because I'll always feel better afterwards.
I have never once worked out & felt worse."
- Alexandra Paul

"The best and most efficient pharmacy
is within your own system."
- Robert C. Peale

"You can be a victim of cancer,
or a survivor of cancer.
It's a mindset."
- Dave Pelzer

"You pray for good health and a
body that will be strong in old age.
Good - but your rich foods block the gods' answer
and tie Jupiter's hands."
- Persius

"I always advise eating regular meals -
a mix of healthy carbs, protein and fruits and veggies."
- Gunnar Peterson

"I am a big believer in taking
responsibility for your actions.
I tell my kids every day to 'own it' -
'it' being whatever they've said or done.
At some point in your life, you are in charge.
You call the shots. You decide to eat or not eat.
Is lack of will power a disease?
Is lack of self-discipline a disease?
I would love to eat my body weight in chocolate chip cookies,
french fries, and peanut butter, but I don't. I choose not to.
That's on me, just like it's on me if I choose to do it."
- Gunnar Peterson

"I think the AMA got this one wrong
(labeling Obesity a 'disease')
and I think the repercussions are going to be ugly.
America wasn't made on blame; it was made on responsibility.
Take off the training wheels in life and
decide to take responsibility for your actions."
- Gunnar Peterson

"Cancer is that awful word we all fear
when we go to the doctor for a physical exam,
but in that brief dark moment we hear it
the world we live in and the people we share it with
begin to illuminate things we did not even pay attention to."
- BD Phillips

"Youth has no age."
- Pablo Picasso

"Happiness is the true goal behind the things we do.
Don't ever let people hijack this goal from you."
- Brad Pilon

"I think the very point is
to not let things like TV distract us.
So eat when hungry, not eat when bored.
Go to sleep when tired,
not go to sleep when American Idol is over."
- Brad Pilon

"Attention to health is life's greatest hindrance."
- Plato

"Lack of activity destroys the
good condition of every human being,
while movement and methodical physical exercise
save it and preserve it."
- Plato

"Every major food company
now has an organic division.
There's more capital going into
organic agriculture
than ever before."
- Michael Pollan

"It's not food if it arrived
through the window of your car."
- Michael Pollan

"Very simply, we subsidize high-fructose corn syrup
in this country, but not carrots.
While the surgeon general is raising alarms
over the epidemic of obesity,
the president is signing farm bills designed to
keep the river of cheap corn flowing,
guaranteeing that the cheapest calories
in the supermarket will continue to be the unhealthiest."
- Michael Pollan

"It's been said that people become like their friends,
loved ones, and associates (and even their pets!).
If you want to be healthy, you should hang out
with healthy people and absorb their energy.
If you want to be happy, you should
surround yourself with happy people."
- Chris Powell

"Small changes over time lead
to extraordinary long-term results!"
- Chris Powell

"The chief condition on which, life, health
and vigor depend on is action.
It is by action that an organism develops its faculties,
increases its energy, and
attains the fulfillment of its destiny."
- Colin Powell

"Get Moving Tip: Before going to bed,
leave your running shoes on
your bathroom counter (or throw them in your gym bag!)
so they're the first thing you see in the morning.
Sometimes, that extra reminder to
get moving is the best motivator!"
- Heidi Powell

"As long as my body is in shape,
my mind is working at its full capacity."
- Victoria Principal

"I believe that how you feel is very important to how you look
- that healthy equals beautiful."
- Victoria Principal

"It is so easy to forget that this is good that we're alive.
We should be enjoying this gift of being alive."
- Victoria Principal

"A healthy human body is self regulating and self repairing."
- Patricia Quillan

"There is an abundance of scientific evidence
showing that a clinically guided nutrition program
for the cancer patient can
improve quality of life by 12 to 21 fold...
and a greater likelihood of complete remission."
- Patrick Quillin

"I'm nutty for nutrition. I've become one of those
people who can't stop talking about the
connection between food and health.
Now that I know how much changing what you eat
can transform your life, I can't stop proselytizing."
- Robin Quivers

"I started running 3 miles every morning after throat surgery
to remove a cyst last year.
The gym used to be my adversary.
But that has all changed.
Now, I look forward to it every morning."
- Rachael Ray

"I've never been a huge sweets eater,
and I've always loved a Mediterranean diet.
We eat a lot of dark leafy greens,
and a couple meals each week are meat-free.
We enjoy eating a balanced diet."
- Rachael Ray

"You can't 'take' a breath,
your breath is given to you."
- Shiva Rea

"Courage is not the absence of fear,
but rather the judgment that
something else is more important than fear."
- Ambrose Redmoon

"Once you choose hope,
anything's possible."
- Christopher Reeve

"The patient should be made to understand that
he or she must take charge of his own life.
Don't take your body to the doctor
as if he were a repair shop."
- Quentin Regestein

"No one is immune from obesity - it affects
everyone from every race, gender and age.
For the first time in history,
there is a real possibility that children
will not outlive their parents as a result of
weight-related illnesses and other diseases.
There has to be a better way!"
- Tosca Reno

"Put simply, Clean Eating
is avoiding all processed food,
relying on fresh fruits, vegetables and
whole grains rather than prepackaged or fast food."
- Tosca Reno

"Remember that a healthy body is built or destroyed
one decision at a time. It's up to you."
- Tosca Reno

"Some of the most challenging moves towards health
are made with the simplest of steps and that is why
I wrote 'The Start Here Diet'."
- Tosca Reno

"As places of learning,
schools have a responsibility
to also educate on nutrition,
which we all can agree is
far more important than algebra,
no matter what your third-period teacher claims."
- Lynda Resnick

"There is so much medical evidence
to support oxygen therapies
that no media dared cover it."
- Duncan Rhoads

"Awareness is bad for the meat business.
Conscience is bad for the meat business.
Sensitivity to life is bad for the meat business.
DENIAL however,
the meat business finds indispensable."
- John Robbins

"Few of us are aware that the act of eating
can be a powerful statement of commitment
to our own well-being, and at the same time the
creation of a healthier habitat.
Your health, happiness, and the
future of life on earth are
rarely so much in your own hands
as when you sit down to eat."
- John Robbins

"I believe that eating simple food in a healthy body
with a clean conscience is more pleasurable,
and infinitely more satisfying,
then eating decadent food
that makes you and your world ill."
- John Robbins

"The fork is the most powerful tool
ever placed in our hands."
- John Robbins

"The joy is that we can take back our bodies,
reclaim our health, and restore ourselves to balance.
We can take power over what and how we eat.
We can rejuvenate and recharge ourselves,
bringing healing to the wounds we carry inside us,
and bringing to fuller life the
wonderful person that each of us can be."
- John Robbins

"You know that a majority of the medical costs
that are bankrupting families, companies,
and nations could be eliminated with better nutrition."
- John Robbins

"There is a reason why more
than forty insurance companies
now cover all or part of the Ornish program.
Nearly 80 percent of patients with severely
clogged arteries who follow the Ornish program
for a year or more are able to avoid bypass or angioplasty.
Despite (or maybe because of) such outstanding results,
the Ornish program has been the subject of massive controversy.
Some say his approach is too drastic,
and we should stick to more medically conservative methods.
Ornish's reply is simple and difficult to argue with:
'I don't understand why asking people to eat
a well-balanced vegetarian diet is considered drastic,
while it's medically conservative to cut people open or put them
on powerful cholesterol-lowering drugs for the rest of their lives'."
- John Robbins

"Cut down on animal products.
Approximately one-third of the calories consumed
by people living in developed nations are from animal sources.
Animal foods - like meat, poultry, fish, milk, and cheese
are usually an expensive source of protein and nutrients."
- Ocean Robbins

"Grow food. It takes time, but gardening is the
most economical way to enjoy the freshest possible food."
- Ocean Robbins

"Healthy food is a fundamental building block for a healthy life."
- Ocean Robbins

"Alkalize and Energize!"
- Tony Robbins

"Motion creates emotion."
- Tony Robbins

"Now, more than ever, busy lifestyles, stress,
easy access to fast foods,
exposure to toxic chemicals,
and a diminished quality of our food supply
require that we take control
and actively pursue the health, energy
and vitality we all desire and deserve now."
- Tony Robbins

"Nothing tastes as good as excellent health."
- Tony Robbins

"Science has now proven that
how you think about stress matters
- the story you attach to stress.
Telling yourself it's good for you instead of harmful
could mean the difference between a
stress-induced heart attack at 50
or living well into your 90s."
- Tony Robbins

"The only people without problems are those in cemeteries."
- Tony Robbins

"The quality of your life is dependent upon the
quality of the life of your cells.
If the bloodstream is filled with waste products,
the resulting environment does not promote a strong, vibrant,
healthy cell life-or biochemistry capable of
creating a balanced emotional life for an individual."
- Tony Robbins

"Want to learn to eat a lot?
Here it is: Eat a little.
That way, you will be around long enough to eat a lot."
- Tony Robbins

"Every now and again I just really have to have that
steak or lamb chop. But yeah, B.C. (before cancer)
I would eat red meat probably
three or four times a week, easily.
I am convinced that the amount
of red meat I ate contributed to it."
- Robin Roberts

"Everything's the same;
I'm living with cancer and it's not going to stop me.
But until you really test yourself
and challenge yourself,
I don't think you quite know."
- Robin Roberts

"It's about focusing on the fight and not the fright."
- Robin Roberts

"It was part of the reason I almost
didn't go public with my diagnosis
- I was embarrassed.
I felt, 'Oh, I've always talked about exercising.
And I got cancer.' And then I realized
it's a great example of showing that
cancer can hit anyone at any time."
- Robin Roberts

"I've still got it. I refuse to lose."
- Robin Roberts

"Take care of your body.
It's the only place you have to live."
- Jim Rohn

"Four studies, all reported in the last five years,
have found what many suspected all along:
that a positive attitude makes a large difference
in how long and how well you live."
- Michael F. Roizen

"If any food has any one of the five ingredients
below as any one of the first five
ingredients on the label,
don't let it near your mouth.
1) Simple sugars
2) Enriched, bleached, or refined flour
(this means it's stripped of its nutrients)
3) All syrups, including HFCS
(high-fructose corn syrup - a four-letter word)
4) Saturated fat
(four legged animal fat or palm or coconut oil)
5) Trans fat
(partially hydrogenated vegetable oil)."
- Michael F. Roizen

"In fact, behavioral choices account almost entirely for
a person's overall health and longevity by age sixty.
The older you are, the more your choices determine
how long and how well you live."
- Michael F. Roizen

"To help curb hunger and avoid binge eating,
drink a glass or two of water before you eat."
- Michael F. Roizen

"Walk thirty minutes a day and build a little muscle.
When you lose some weight,
your cells become more sensitive
and responsive to leptin."
- Michael F. Roizen

"A big barrier to getting people to
eat more fruits and vegetables is
convenience, the packaging and accessibility."
- Barbara Rolls

"I think it's quite obvious we need
innovative strategies to limit the
impact of portion size on intake."
- Barbara Rolls

"People like value. We've got to shift people
away from this value way of thinking
of simply getting the most
calories for the least dollars,
to value in terms of health."
- Barbara Rolls

"Be consistent:
It's not about how much you do
in a given workout or how hard it is.
Ten minutes of core exercises four to five times
per week is far better
than one long run a week."
- Rich Roll

"Don't diet:
Instead, get honest about your habits
and embark on implementing healthy,
lasting changes in your nutrition.
I feel quite strongly that a nutrition program
built entirely around plant-based foods
and completely devoid of
animal products is optimal."
- Rich Roll

"It's crazy how emotional and threatened people
can become when the subject turns to food and diet.
Merely mentioning plant-based nutrition
often prompts immediate debate.
But I relish the dialogue.
It's been a kick confronting
head-on the arguments of the critics
and dissenting voices and putting them to the test.
I've done my homework. I know how I feel.
And my results speak for themselves."
- Rich Roll

"Let's join together to shift the world's perspective
on long-term health and wellness.
No matter how old, overweight or out of shape you are,
you have the power to make a decision,
set a goal and create a plan.
Positive change is always within your grasp,
and today still remains the first day of the rest of your life.
Make it count!"
- Rich Roll

"Let's wrap up the protein question
with one thought to ponder.
Some of the strongest and most fierce animals
in the world are Plant Powered.
The elephant, rhino, hippo, and gorilla
have one thing in common -
they all get 100 percent of their protein from plants."
- Rich Roll

"Nothing changes if nothing changes."
- Rich Roll

"Remember that it's not about the result
- it's about the journey."
- Rich Roll

"The prize never goes to the fastest guy.
It goes to the guy who slows down the least.
True in endurance sports.
And possibly even truer in life."
- Rich Roll

"When the mind is controlled and spirit aligned with purpose,
the body is capable of so much more than we realize."
- Rich Roll

"Buy the jeans that make your ass look the nicest."
- John Romaniello

"Floss your teeth for better fitness."
- John Romaniello

"Learn how to cook.
If you're approaching 30 and you
can't make a few meals,
take the next month and learn."
- John Romaniello

"Of all the people on the planet,
you talk to yourself more than anyone.
Make sure you are saying the right things."
- Martin Rooney

"You gain strength, courage, and confidence by every experience
in which you really stop to look fear in the face.
You must do the thing which you think you cannot do."
- Eleanor Roosevelt

"When you come to the end of your rope, tie a knot and hang on."
- Franklin D. Roosevelt

"You will know if you are too acidic if you get sick often,
get urinary tract infections, suffer from headaches,
and have bad breath and body odor
(when you do not use antiperspirant).
Acidosis is the medical term for
a blood alkalinity of less than 7.35.
A normal reading is called homeostasis.
It is not considered a disease;
although in and of itself it is
recognized as an indicator of disease."
- Natalia Rose

"Being lean is not normal in today's society.
This means you need to do things that normal people don't do.
You need to pack your own lunch;
you need to request food be prepared
differently than what's listed on most menus;
your idea of 'fast food' should be a protein shake; and you
can't take the weekend off from your diet like you do your job."
- Mike Roussell

"Nowadays everyone is connected every second of everyday.
Cell phones, internet, email, TiVo, you know what I mean.
It is so important to unplug yourself.
Meditation is another great way to reduce stress and cortisol.
You don't have to become a monk or
anything but 20 minutes of sitting with no distractions
and focusing on your breathing will do wonders."
- Mike Roussell

"70% of long-term gym memberships are mostly unused,
but a dog needs walking every day."
- Gretchen Rubin

"I should make one healthy choice,
and then stop choosing."
- Gretchen Rubin

"Once the habit is in place,
we can effortlessly do the things we want to do."
- Gretchen Rubin

"The desire to start something at the 'right' time
is usually just a justification for delay.
In almost every case, the best time to start is now."
- Gretchen Rubin

"What you do every day matters more
than what you do once in a while."
- Gretchen Rubin

"Emotional health is critical."
- Jordan Rubin

"Hypertension is only a symptom of some
other malfunction in your body.
It's possible that the elevated blood pressure is a protective effect,
enabling the heart to get blood to all the tissues in spite of
the disease, whatever that might be.
But since we still haven't figured out what that reason is,
most physicians just throw drugs at the symptom and consider
the problem solved when the high blood pressure goes down."
- Jordan Rubin

"My private measure of success is daily.
If this were to be the last day of my life
would I be content with it?
To live in a harmonious balance of commitments
and pleasures is what I strive for."
- Jane Rule

"Don't grieve. Anything you lose comes round in another form."
- Rumi

"Everything in the universe is within you.
Ask all from yourself."
- Rumi

"I am not this hair,
I am not this skin,
I am the soul that lives within."
- Rumi

"Ignore those that make you fearful and sad,
that degrade you back towards disease and death."
- Rumi

"The cure for pain is in the pain."
- Rumi

"Yesterday I was clever, so I wanted to change the world.
Today I am wise, so I am changing myself."
- Rumi

"Motivation is what gets you started.
Habit is what keeps you going."
- Jim Ryun

"Trust me if you're sick, it's not because
you're pharmaceutically disadvantaged."
- Joel Salatin

"I was a vegetarian first.
I had high blood pressure at 27,
everybody in my family died of cancer,
and I knew it was in the food,
so I changed my diet."
- John Salley

"Children want to mimic adults.
They notice when you choose to prepare
fresh vegetables over calling in
another pizza pie for dinner.
They will see that food made with love and care
outweighs going through the drive-through window."
- Marcus Samuelsson

"Let the fresh fruits and vegetables be your guide,
and make something that will keep for the whole week."
- Marcus Samuelsson

"I was a vegan for two years, and I really enjoyed it.
Then, I got to a point in my life at which I wanted
to do something else, so now I'm a vegetarian.
You should make your diet one that best fits you
and how you feel. Listen to your body.
The most important thing is to exercise,
drink lots of water, and
take really good care of yourself."
- Lea Michele Sarfati (aka Lea Michele)

"Looking after my health today gives me
a better hope for tomorrow."
- Anne Wilson Schaef

"We have finally started to notice that
there is real curative value in local herbs
and remedies. In fact, we are also
becoming aware that there are little or no
side effects to most natural remedies,
and that they are often more
effective than Western medicine."
- Anne Wilson Schaef

"We are basically overloaded with all the
health information coming our way.
I like to go back to basics. Detoxification first,
then boosting the immune system with
concentrated and nutrient dense drinks and foods.
We don't need much, but we do need the best possible
foods and some supplements, such as green power foods
- algae, spirulina, wheat grass and others. We need a plan.
We need direction and encouragement, purpose and hope."
- Jill Schneider

"The greatest of follies is to sacrifice health
for any other kind of happiness."
- Arthur Schopenhauer

"Doctors said 'go home and enjoy what little is left of your life'.
He recovered."
- Richard Schulze

"Garlic has been shown to help our white blood cells
not only defend us against cancer, but also to increase our ability
to destroy tumors...Garlic has been found to stimulate interferon
production, enhance natural killer cells, stop tumor growth,
and even reduce the associated pain of cancer.
Most of the research has been done
on cancers of the digestive tract."
- Richard Schulze

"My parents both had heart disease. They were under complete
medical doctors' care. They were allowed to smoke cigarettes, drink
pots of coffee and excessive alcohol, consume outrageous amounts
of sugar and live on a diet of almost pure animal fat, have a bowel
movement once a week or less, never exercise, and were directed
to take a dozen toxic, chemical pharmaceutical drugs
to try and offset their toxic and lethal lifestyle.
This medical program didn't work out for them..."
- Richard Schulze

"Natural healing has the power to cure pancreatic cancer.
But usually, before I see the patient, medical treatments
- not the disease have destroyed the patient's body."
- Richard Schulze

"The famous herbalist Samuel Thompson
used two herbs mainly, cayenne & lobelia.
And with those two herbs, it is estimated he
helped 3.5 million people recover from their illnesses."
- Richard Schulze

"The man's prostate was so encased by
the tumour that doctors couldn't even see it.
The tumour was wrapped around the gland...
when he started out his PSA was around 5,000...
it eventually normalised...and he is alive and well now...
and I think his PSA count is like 3 or 4."
- Richard Schulze

"With every episode of struggle,
there is a learning opportunity."
- Richard Schulze

"You can heal yourself of ANYTHING,
any illness or dis-ease.
Just STOP doing what made you sick, and
START doing what will Create Powerful Health.
There are NO incurable diseases, NONE.
Take RESPONSIBILITY, and be willing to CHANGE,
and you can heal yourself of anything."
- Richard Schulze

"I'm addicted to exercising and
I have to do something every day."
- Arnold Schwarzenegger

"Strength does not come from winning.
Your struggles develop your strengths.
When you go through hardships
and decide not to surrender,
that is strength."
- Arnold Schwarzenegger

"The resistance that you fight physically in the gym
and the resistance that you fight in life
can only build a strong character."
- Arnold Schwarzenegger

"What we face may look insurmountable.
But I learned something from all those years
of training and competing.
I learned something from all those sets and reps
when I didn't think I could lift another ounce of weight.
What I learned is that we are
always stronger than we know."
- Arnold Schwarzenegger

"The human spirit is stronger
than anything that can happen to it."
- C.C. Scott

"What's the whole point of being pretty on the
outside when you're so ugly on the inside?"
- Jess C. Scott

"What makes me so certain that the natural
human lifespan is far in excess of the actual one is this.
Among all my autopsies (and I have performed over 1,000),
I have never seen a person who died of old age.
In fact, I do not think that anyone has ever died of old age yet."
- Hans Selye

"The wish for healing has
always been half of health."
- Lucius Annaeus Seneca

"Wherever there is a human being,
there is an opportunity for kindness."
- Lucius Annaeus Seneca

"Most people don't have a problem going on a diet.
Their problem is being consistent on their diet."
- Karen Sessions

"Processed foods not only extend the shelf life,
but they extend the waistline as well."
- Karen Sessions

"Our bodies are our gardens
- our wills are our gardeners."
- William Shakespeare

"Eat real food at least 90% of the time."
- Nia Shanks

"It's more important that you develop habits
that are easy to maintain over a longer period of time
as opposed to employing a drastic change overnight."
- Nia Shanks

"Use your health,
even to the point of wearing it out.
That is what it is for.
Spend all you have before you die;
do not outlive yourself."
- George Bernard Shaw

"We don't stop playing because we grow old;
we grow old because we stop playing."
- George Bernard Shaw

"Because of physicians' limited medical training,
rarely do we have the option to learn
about the true cause of disease.
And yet it is possible to prevent disease
and emotional breakdown."
- Bernie S. Siegel

"I began to realize a patient's beliefs
were more important than the diagnosis."
- Bernie S. Siegel

"If you talk to your body, it will listen."
- Bernie S. Siegel

"I know patients who bring a dozen roses to the doctor's office.
And, boy, the next visit, nobody forgets that.
You come in and hey -
'Here's the lady who brought the roses'
vs. 'Here's the lung cancer'."
- Bernie S. Siegel

"Inspiration is the greatest gift because
it opens your life to many new possibilities.
Each day becomes more meaningful,
and your life is enhanced when
your actions are guided by what inspires you."
- Bernie S. Siegel

"I was not a typical surgeon, because I kept
trying to help my patients in nontraditional ways."
- Bernie S. Siegel

"Laughter is one of the best therapeutic activities
Mother Nature provides us with, and it doesn't cost a cent."
- Bernie S. Siegel

"Most of us never stop to consider our blessings;
rather, we spend the day only thinking about our problems.
But since you have to be alive to have problems,
be grateful for the opportunity to have them."
- Bernie S. Siegel

"One of the best ways to change is to act
as if you are the person you want to become.
When you behave as if you are a different person,
you change on a very basic level
- even your physiology changes.
When actors and actresses perform,
their body chemistry is altered by the roles they play."
- Bernie S. Siegel

"Parents, teachers, clergy and physicians
change lives with their words.
It is hypnotic for a child or patient
to hear an authority figure's words.
As I am always sharing, 'wordswordswords'
can become 'swordswordswords,'
and we can kill or cure with either words or swords."
- Bernie S. Siegel

"People can be talked into health or illness."
- Bernie S. Siegel

"Physicians are not taught how to communicate with patients.
Because of their fear of being sued,
they tell people about all the adverse side effects
of therapy and never mention the benefits."
- Bernie S. Siegel

"The need for encouraging more
of a mind-body-spirit approach
in medicine is still great, especially
in the training of medical professionals."
- Bernie S. Siegel

"Scientists have studied the effects
of laughter on the body and identified
a number of physiological benefits.
Laughter increases activity in the immune system,
giving 'good' killer cells a boost,
especially in their ability to target viruses,
some tumors, and cancer cells."
- Bernie S. Siegel

"The doctor I would want for myself or for anyone else
I cared about would be one who understands
that disease is more than just a clinical entity;
it is an experience and a metaphor,
with a message that must be listened to."
- Bernie S. Siegel

"The mind and body are not separate units,
but one integrated system.
How we act and what we think, eat,
and feel are all related to our health.
Physicians should be capable of
teaching this behavior to patients."
- Bernie S. Siegel

"Today we have studies documenting that
cancer patients who laughed or practiced
induced laughter several times a day
lived longer than a control group who did not."
- Bernie S. Siegel

"Whatever we imagine, and what we focus on,
sends a message to our body,
so when we draw healing images
our body follows through."
- Bernie S. Siegel

"When lifestyle counseling was incorporated into the
medical treatment plan for patients with advanced cancer,
their survival time doubled and their quality of life improved."
- Bernie S. Siegel

"When you love your life and body,
your body will do all it can to keep you alive."
- Bernie S. Siegel

"You can't control the world, but
when you control your thoughts, you bring order."
- Bernie S. Siegel

"Your thoughts and feelings
create your internal chemistry."
- Bernie S. Siegel

"He who laughs, lasts."
- Bobbie S. Siegel

"Cancer changes your life, often for the better.
You learn what's important, you learn to prioritize,
and you learn not to waste your time.
You tell people you love them. My friend Gilda Radner
used to say, 'If it wasn't for the downside,
having cancer would be the best thing
and everyone would want it.'
That's true. If it wasn't for the downside."
- Joel Siegel

"Do what will make you happy."
- Rose Siegel

"Sickness is the vengeance of nature
for the violation of her laws."
- Charles Simmons

"For my workout, I'm up at 4 am
I say my prayers, count my blessings,
and I work out right away. I just get it done."
- Richard Simmons

"If you pick up every other magazine,
it is the peanut butter diet,
or the cabbage soup diet,
and then you go to the radio and you
hear that you can drink some solution
and you will lose weight overnight.
It just does not work that way!"
- Richard Simmons

"I've always practiced this:
Love yourself. Move your body. Watch your portions."
- Richard Simmons

"I have rules about eating, exercising and
rules about staying positive.
And these rules are sacred to me."
- Richard Simmons

"No tricks, gimmicks, special pills,
special potions, special equipment.
All it takes is desire and will."
- Richard Simmons

"If you wake up deciding what you want to give
versus what you're going to get,
you become a more successful person."
- Russell Simmons

"I go to yoga every day.
I meditate every morning."
- Russell Simmons

"I mostly eat healthy. I just do.
I'm not a vegan for health reasons -
although I'm 20 pounds lighter than when I started.
I stayed 20 pounds lighter. I feel better.
My friends say I look better. All that's true.
But I'm a vegan for compassionate reasons."
- Russell Simmons

"You can learn to follow the inner self,
the inner physician that tells you where to go.
Healing is simply attempting to do more of those things
that bring joy and fewer of those things that bring pain."
- O. Carl Simonton

"The question you need to ask yourself is
not if you will heal, but how you will heal."
- O. Carl Simonton

"When you're depressed,
the whole body is depressed,
and it translates to the cellular level.
The first objective is to get your energy up,
and you can do it through play.
It's one of the most powerful ways of breaking up
Hopelessness and bringing energy into the situation."
- O. Carl Simonton

"A doctor has to speak in positives.
If a doctor puts out negative energy,
the patients will take it in unconsciously."
- Stephen Sinatra

"The most important thing I can instill into the patient
is the belief that he or she can get well."
- Stephen Sinatra

"Eliminating grains and sugars from your diet
could be the number one most beneficial thing
you ever do for your health!"
- Mark Sisson

"Our government's laws, subsidies, and diet education efforts
are seemingly driven more by lobbyists for the
beef, grain, and dairy industries than by unbiased
scientific evaluation and concern for human health."
- Mark Sisson

"Reduced Disease Risk Factors:
Ditching grains, sugars, other simple carbs,
and processed foods, especially 'bad fats'
(trans and partially-hydrogenated),
will reduce your production of hormone-like
messengers that instruct genes to make
harmful pro-inflammatory protein agents.
These agents increase your risk for arthritis, diabetes,
cancer, heart disease, and many other
inflammation-related health problems."
- Mark Sisson

"Studies suggest that overweight kids are highly likely
to become overweight adults and consequently suffer
from serious health problems and life-threatening diseases."
- Mark Sisson

"Those who think they have no time for healthy eating,
will sooner or later have to find time for illness."
- Edward Stanley

"Those who do not find time for exercise
will have to find time for illness."
- Edward Stanley

"It's bizarre that the produce manager is more important
to my children's health than the pediatrician."
- Meryl Streep

"The important thing is not how many years in your life
but how much life in your years."
- Edward J. Stieglitz

"Have you ever noticed how there is always some new food
that is being 'discovered' for its mystical healing properties?
Every year it seems like there is another fad food that people
will flock to for a little while before they go back to eating
the way they have all their lives."
- Kimberly Snyder

"How close is the food to its natural state?
What sort of process did it undergo to wind up
in that package at the grocery store?"
- Kimberly Snyder

"I believe the word 'health' is
synonymous with the word beauty.
My definition of beauty is that
it's deep, lasting, and magnetic,
and it grows from the inside out."
- Kimberly Snyder

"That step of picking up your own food will
cut out more and more processed foods."
- Kimberly Snyder

"We are the only species on earth that
not only refuses to give up milk but furthermore
insists on drinking the milk of another species.
No adult cows ever drink milk,
and adult humans are certainly
not meant to be drinking it, either!
As is always the case,
when we go against nature's laws,
we suffer the consequences."
- Kimberly Snyder

"Why is it that two people get coughed on
directly in the face (gross!) by the same person
on the subway, but only one person gets the flu?
Dr. Robert Young gives a great analogy
to this by pointing out that if you throw
seeds on concrete, they cannot grow.
But if you throw the seeds on fertile soil,
they grow and flourish.
And so it is with germs and sickness."
- Kimberly Snyder

"Every chemical that makes it into your bloodstream
- be it through your lungs, stomach, or skin
meets up with your liver at some point.
Since your liver is your body's best defense
when it comes to filtering out all those toxins,
you need to treat it well."
- Suzanne Somers

"Forgiveness is a gift you give yourself."
- Suzanne Somers

"I am not a doctor or a scientist, but merely
a passionate layperson, a filter, a messenger.
I spoke with so many patients who are living normal, happy,
fulfilled lives, and their enthusiasm and great quality of life
convinced me that you can indeed live with cancer."
- Suzanne Somers

"I am healthy;
it is the greatest gift I have given myself."
- Suzanne Somers

"I am in control of how I age, and I am in control of my health."
- Suzanne Somers

"I appreciate health care that gets to the root cause
of our symptoms and promotes wellness, rather than
the one-size-fits-all drug-based approach to treating disease.
I love maintaining an optimal quality of life - naturally."
- Suzanne Somers

"I'm going to live to be 110 years old!"
- Suzanne Somers

"It is a very brave choice to go against
traditional medicine and embrace the alternative route.
It's easier to try the traditional route and then, if it fails,
go to the alternatives, but often it can be too late."
- Suzanne Somers

"I would like to do my own daily talk show.
Wisdom is the gift of aging; no young person can have or buy it.
My success was and is self-evident. I'm alive. I've lived.
I've thrived and have grown as a person.
I'm now healthier than ever. Who can argue with that?"
- Suzanne Somers

"The biggest myth about aging is
that we can't do anything about it.
That it's a road to being decrepit, frail, and sick."
- Suzanne Somers

"We stopped cleaning our houses with
lemon water and vinegar like our mothers did,
and we clean with chemicals.
We're breathing chemicals, and then
everyone wonders why cancer is the biggest killer."
- Suzanne Somers

"When you receive a cancer diagnosis,
you're more vulnerable than at any other time in your life.
I've personally had the experience twice.
My only hope for survival was alternatives.
But that was my decision,
what I thought was best for me."
- Suzanne Somers

"You can manage cancer.
You don't have to be degraded
by humiliating treatments and protocols.
And in some cases, you can be cured of cancer."
- Suzanne Somers

"Heart disease continues to be the number one killer;
cancer, the number 2 killer, not far behind.
The tragic aspect of these deadly diseases
is that they could all be cured,
I do believe, if we had sufficient funding."
- Arlen Specter

"The best way to reduce the cost of medical care
is to reduce the illness."
- Arlen Specter

"There's nothing more important than our good health
- that's our principal capital asset."
- Arlen Specter

"Those who think they have not time for bodily exercise
will sooner or later have to find time for illness."
- Lord Edward Stanley

"Looking good and feeling good go hand in hand.
If you have a healthy lifestyle, your diet and nutrition are set,
and you're working out, you're going to feel good."
- Jason Statham

"It's not enough to exercise. You have got to sleep.
You have got to drink enough water.
You have got to develop a practice
around maintenance of your body.
You have got to learn how to move right."
- Kelly Starrett

"One of the things I do to stay healthy and fit
is to make sure I exercise every single day.
Aside from eating right and getting enough sleep,
exercise keeps me trim and boosts my energy."
- Martha Stewart

"You can be the most beautiful person on Earth,
and if you don't have a fitness or diet routine,
you won't be beautiful."
- Martha Stewart

"I grow my own vegetables and herbs.
I like being able to tell people that the lunch
I'm serving started out as a seed in my yard."
- Curtis Stone

"You've got to set yourself up to be as healthy as you can.
The thing we tend to do is when it gets to be a bit too hard,
actually opt out for the absolute worst option.
For example, if you're in a rush in a morning
and you feel like you don't have time
to make breakfast, you skip it."
- Curtis Stone

"Deprivation doesn't work for me,
and research shows it doesn't work
for most other people, either."
- Travis Stork

"Every time you sit down to eat,
you are making a life-changing decision.
You are deciding how well you want to live.
You are deciding how long you want to live.
And you are deciding how good you want to feel,
today and for the rest of your life.
In fact, every time you even look at a piece of food,
you are gazing at the destiny of your health."
- Travis Stork

"Focus on flavor, because life is too short to eat tasteless food!"
- Travis Stork

"No matter how bad your diet is,
no matter how much excess weight you're carrying around,
no matter how many food-related mistakes
you've made in the past, you can start fresh now."
- Travis Stork

"The biggest emergency in ERs across the United States
is the food we willingly, knowingly, happily choose to eat."
- Travis Stork

"First and Foremost, our food should be healthy.
Food is medicine. It can kill.
It can cure. It's THAT powerful."
- Rob Sulaver

"I'm not saying NEVER indulge.
I'm saying, indulge intelligently.
Ideal nutrition strikes a perfect balance of
short and long term satisfaction.
It's your body and you're gonna have to live in it tomorrow.
That's why optimal nutrition isn't perfect.
It's balanced: Usually awesome.
Sometimes guilty. Occasionally downright glutenous.
Make the right choice 85% of the time and you're
well on your way to a solid nutrition plan."
- Rob Sulaver

"The food we consume should make us strong, capable,
and energized for whatever we do."
- Rob Sulaver

"Why are vegetables so damn good for us?
The vitamins and minerals in vegetables
are exceptionally bioavailable.
That means our bodies are very suited to digest and utilize them
('it's not what you eat, it's what you absorb.')
The phytochemicals in vegetables are also powerful anti-oxidants
and have a strong influence on our hormones.
They suppress cancer development,
protect our cell's DNA and stimulate enzymes
that help our body fight disease."
Rob Sulaver

"I started looking for alternative solutions,
because people weren't getting better."
- Murray Susser

"If people are frustrated and have a hunch
that their doctor isn't looking deeply enough
or hearing them well enough,
change doctors.
Also change doctors if a doctor doesn't
want you to have another opinion.
If you're not getting well and your doctor doesn't
want you to have another opinion,
then you need another opinion.
At least that's my feeling."
- Murray Susser

"My approach to patients is one of partnership
in helping with their diseases.
I am the junior partner; the patient is in charge.
I will be the best advisor I can possibly be.
I will offer options, because most of the things
that I do don't have rigid protocols."
- Murray Susser

"The immune system plays a pivotal role in cancer;
when the immune system fails for whatever reason,
it may be the reason we get cancer."
- Murray Susser

"When it comes to health, be proactive.
The more proactive a patient is with their health,
the better they do, in my experience."
- Murray Susser

"Good health and good sense
are two of life's greatest blessings."
- Publilius Syrus

"Faith is the bird that feels the light when the dawn is still dark."
- Rabindranath Tagore

"I'm just thankful for everything,
all the blessings in my life, trying to stay that way.
I think that's the best way to
start your day and finish your day.
It keeps everything in perspective."
- Tim Tebow

"I rely on a lot of green drinks to get my vegetables."
- Tim Tebow

"Laughter is important,
not only because it makes us happy,
it also has actual health benefits.
And that's because laughter completely
engages the body and releases the mind.
It connects us to others,
and that in itself has a healing effect.
- Marlo Thomas

"Our body is a machine for living.
It is organized for that, it is its nature.
Let life go on in it unhindered and let it defend itself,
it will do more than if you paralyze it
by encumbering it with remedies."
- Leo Tolstoy

"Just as your car runs more smoothly and requires less energy
to go faster and farther when the wheels are in perfect alignment,
you perform better when your thoughts, feelings,
emotions, goals, and values are in balance."
- Brian Tracy

"Drag your thoughts away from your troubles -
by the ears, by the heels, or any other way, so you manage it;
it's the healthiest thing a body can do."
- Mark Twain

"Worrying about something is like paying interest
on a debt you don't even know you owe".
- Mark Twain

"A healthy outside starts from the inside."
- Robert Urich

"Charge forward with hope and
get the best medical advice you can.
Talk to your friends, neighbors, family,
and together you attack it.
We can't always control what happens to us,
but we can always control how we react to it."
- Robert Urich

"Cancer can take away all of my physical abilities.
It cannot touch my mind, it cannot touch my heart,
and it cannot touch my soul."
- Jim Valvano

"Don't get hung up on the hard times, the challenges.
Tell your story by highlighting the victories.
Because it's your victories that will inspire, motivate, encourage
other people to live their stories in grander ways."
- Iyanla Vanzant

"In my deepest, darkest moments, what really got me through was a
prayer. Sometimes my prayer was 'Help me.' Sometimes a prayer
was 'Thank you.' What I've discovered is that intimate connection
and communication with my creator will always get me through
because I know my support, my help, is just a prayer away."
- Iyanla Vanzant

"I live to save these peoples lives."
- Joseph Vickers

"How can you be a doctor and you get 10 hours of nutrition,
and that's where healing lies? In Chiropractic school,
we got some 160 hours of nutrition while we were in school.
And I studied nutrition like crazy outside of my classes."
- Patrick Vickers

"In 1931, Otto Warburg won the Nobel Prize in medicine when he
was able to prove that viruses, bacteria in cancer cells could not
survive in highly oxygenated environments. That's proof.
That cannot be disputed, that's what he won the Nobel Prize for
back then. And that's exactly why we utilize
oxygen therapy on this protocol."
- Patrick Vickers

"Medical doctors from the day they enter school, literally,
in their first semester of school, they are given a book
that is called 'Quackery in America' and
what do you think that book is comprised of?
It's compromised of all natural therapies."
- Patrick Vickers

"So, how is it that we're able to reverse
all these diseases, not just cancer?
We're reversing virtually every single degenerative disease, whether
it is heart disease, diabetes, lupus, MS, rheumatoid-arthritis."
- Patrick Vickers

"The secret of the Gerson Therapy is the production of energy on a
cellular level. Gerson clearly understood that to rally an immune
system, you had increase the production of energy on a cellular
level in a form what's called ATP. ATP is Adenosine Triphosphate,
it's the energy molecule that the mitochondria produce
inside your cells. When you see someone who is sick and/or dying,
what's one of the first things you notice? They are lethargic.
Why are they lethargic? They are lethargic because they
lost the capacity to produce energy on a cellular level..."
- Patrick Vickers

"When I came across Gerson Therapy, it simplified everything
and put it into a finely made package that truly benefits
a majority of patients that we are dealing with."
- Patrick Vickers

"We don't cure everybody. We don't make that claim.
Some people come to us - their organic systems,
particularly their liver and their kidneys are too far gone to restore.
So we can't heal everybody,
but we heal a lot of people that had been sent home to die.
And those that we can't heal, we extend their lives
significantly and their quality of life."
- Patrick Vickers

"What Gerson discovered, really the secret of the Gerson Therapy,
is the production of energy on a cellular level.
Gerson clearly understood that to rally an immune system,
you had increase the production of energy on a cellular level
in a form what's called ATP (Adenosine Triphosphate),
it's the energy molecule that
the mitochondria produce inside your cells."
- Patrick Vickers

"You can't heal a sick and dying body with poison.
These are bodies that have come to us completely depleted
from years of chemical, emotional, environmental abuse.
And it's depleted organic systems
and weakened them tremendously.
You can't rebuild a body with poison.
There's only one way you can rebuild
a human body and that's pure nutrition and pure detoxification.
And then, on top of that, supplementation, proper supplementation."
- Patrick Vickers

"Don't let your learning lead to knowledge,
let your learning lead to action."
- Tom Venuto

"There's no secret to getting started.
You simply decide and then take your first step.
With each subsequent step, the next one becomes easier..."
- Tom Venuto

"Eat clean food. Drink clean water.
Breathe clean air. Get sunlight."
- Daniel Vitalis

"Happiness cannot be traveled to,
owned, earned, worn or consumed.
Happiness is the spiritual experience of living
every minute with love, grace, and gratitude."
- Denis Waitley

"People who laugh actually live longer
than those who don't laugh.
Few persons realize that health actually
varies according to the amount of laughter."
- James J. Walsh

"Nobody today can say that one does not know
what cancer and its prime cause may be.
On the contrary, there is no disease
whose prime cause is better known,
so that today ignorance is no longer an excuse
that one cannot do more about prevention.
That prevention of cancer will come there is no doubt,
for man wishes to survive.
But how long prevention will be avoided depends
on how long the prophets of agnosticism
will succeed in inhibiting the application of
scientific knowledge in the cancer field.
In the meantime, millions of men
must die of cancer unnecessarily."
- Otto Warburg

"According to Ernest Wynder of the
Sloan-Kettering Institute for Cancer Research
in New York, the time has come when
one can exterminate this kind of cancer
with the help of the active groups
of the respiratory enzymes."
- Otto Warburg

"I began to read and research the known causes of cancer
and learned that environmental toxins,
an unhealthy diet and lifestyle, and stress
were all key health-destroying factors.
I realized that my nutrient-deficient diet of processed food,
fast food, junk food, and factory-farmed animal products
was poisoning and polluting my body.
I also came to understand that my thoughts,
attitudes and emotions were toxic as well."
- Chris Wark

"I decided against chemotherapy.
I chose to overdose on nutrition instead,
giving my body everything it needed to repair,
regenerate, and detoxify.
I immediately adopted a raw vegan diet, eating only fruits,
vegetables, seeds and nuts, and drinking
eight glasses of fresh vegetable juice every day."
- Chris Wark

"I'm not unique, I'm not special, and I'm not the only person
who believes he has healed his own cancer.
There are thousands of us."
- Chris Wark

"Today, over 10 years after my diagnosis,
my wife and I have two beautiful daughters,
I am still cancer-free and in the best physical shape of my life."
- Chris Wark

"Doctors are not allowed to offer any alternative therapies."
- Valerie Warwik

"How can you give poisons to people and expect them to heal?"
- Valerie Warwik

"I was preaching a lot about nutrition and I was
getting looked at like I was a kook."
- Valerie Warwik

"I wasn't even aware as a nurse that they
made money off of chemotherapy."
- Valerie Warwik

"The most powerful thing you can do
is to bring 'healing' to your body."
- Valerie Warwik

"Without your immune system, you don't stand a chance."
- Valerie Warwik

"You can change your diet which will impact
your health far more than anything else."
- Valerie Warwik

"Life is so much brighter when we focus on what matters.
The only way to make sense of change is to plunge into it
flow with it... and join the dance."
- Alan Watts

"Courage is being scared to death...
and saddling up anyway."
- John Wayne

"It would be logical to argue
that in an intact immune system,
there is no room for cancer."
- Bradford S. Weeks

"Fitting a walk into a busy life can be challenging,
so I suggest walking rather driving to work
or to run errands as often as you can
- in other words, think of walking
as alternative transportation."
- Andrew Weil

"Gardening is not trivial.
If you believe that it is,
closely examine why you feel that way.
You may discover that this attitude has been
forced upon you by mass media
and the crass culture it creates and maintains.
The fact is, gardening is just the opposite - it is,
or should be, a central, basic expression of human life."
- Andrew Weil

"Human bodies are designed for regular physical activity.
The sedentary nature of much of modern life
probably plays a significant role
in the epidemic incidence of depression today.
Many studies show that depressed patients who stick
to a regimen of aerobic exercise improve as much
as those treated with medication."
- Andrew Weil

"I am a particular fan of integrative exercise
- that is, exercise that occurs in the course of
doing some productive activity
such as gardening, bicycling to work,
doing home improvement projects and so on."
- Andrew Weil

"I have argued for years that we do not have
a health care system in America.
We have a disease management system
- one that depends on ruinously
expensive drugs and surgeries
that treat health conditions after they manifest
rather than giving our citizens simple diet, lifestyle
and therapeutic tools to keep them healthy."
- Andrew Weil

"It does kids no favors,
and sets them up for a potential lifetime
of poor health and social embarrassment,
to excuse them from family meals of real food.
Everyone benefits from healthy eating,
but it is particularly crucial at the beginning of life."
- Andrew Weil

"Technology has a shadow side.
It accounts for real progress in medicine,
but has also hurt it in many ways,
making it more impersonal, expensive and dangerous.
The false belief that a safety net of
sophisticated drugs and machines stretches below us,
permitting risky or lazy lifestyle choices,
has undermined our spirit of self-reliance."
- Andrew Weil

"A man's health can be judged by which he takes
two at a time - pills or stairs."
- Joan Welsh

"Note that the two physicians in
our sampling elected not to be treated
with radiation or chemotherapy."
- Virginia Livingston Wheeler

"We know that conventional therapy doesn't work
- if it did you would not fear cancer any more
than you fear pneumonia.
It is the utter lack of certainty as
to the outcome of conventional treatment
that virtually screams for more freedom of choice
in the area of cancer therapy.
Yet most so-called alternative therapies regardless
of potential or proven benefit, are outlawed,
which forces patients to submit to the failures
we know don't work, because there is no other choice."
- Julian Whitaker

"The most important step for the human body
is daily gentle detoxification."
- Darrell Wolfe

"As a building biologist,
the first thing you want to do
is remove the source of the problem.
It's the same thing we do in holistic health,
remove the source of the problem.
We can actually use what I call holistic bandages,
but it gets back to your daily routine.
Is that daily routine supporting
the human cell, its functionality?
If it is, then you're going to be a healthy person."
- Marcel Wolfe

"Chlorophyll has a frequency. A plant, an apple
that we pick from the tree has its
highest frequency and that is why this whole
fresh and raw movement is so huge.
Because the energy can be measured and it is higher
than if we transport that fruit or vegetable
from Mexico to Canada, nuke it, whatever."
- Marcel Wolfe

"If you've got cancer,
you are going to want to
put all of your options in your favor.
You're going to want to eat the food
with the highest frequency,
drink the water with the highest frequency,
and sleep in a bed that is not metal,
that you don't have the cordless phone
and the cell phone on your pillow,
and all these crazy things.
You need to become more mindful
about what you're doing in
your life to enhance your opportunity
and your children's opportunity
to have the best life possible."
- Marcel Wolfe

"As a society, we have become
so sick, weak, and broken,
we accept the abnormal as normal."
- Robb Wolf

"Exercise is important, but diet is critical."
- Robb Wolf

"If you are concerned about skin cancer
because of this sun exposure,
keep in mind, safe, incremental sun exposure
(not burning your skin)
decreases your likelihood of developing a
host of cancers far more than it increases
your likelihood of developing skin cancer."
- Robb Wolf

"The interior of the grocery store is your foe,
unless you're buying detergent, coffee, or cat litter."
- Robb Wolf

"The United States is in a
health care crisis, the economy is shaky,
and the government subsidizes the production of corn,
making high-fructose corn syrup cheaper than dirt.
Processed food manufacturers make crap foods that
are making us sick, diabetic, and dead too early.
The government subsidizes the development
of statins and a host of drugs to
manage the diseases that are a direct outgrowth
of the processed foods they are subsidizing!"
- Robb Wolf

"Worst-case scenario:
You spend a month without some foods you like.
Best-case scenario:
You discover you are able to live healthier and
better than you ever thought possible."
- Robb Wolf

"There are many things that are essential
to arriving at true peace of mind,
and one of the most important is faith,
which cannot be acquired without prayer."
- John Wooden

"Things turn out best for people who make
the best of the way things turn out."
- John Wooden

"If you live right, the cancer will never ever
manifest itself in your body."
- Bob Wright

"Lifestyle can totally change gene expression".
- Bob Wright

"No doctor has ever healed anyone of
anything in the history of the world.
The human immune system heals
and that's the only thing that heals."
- Bob Wright

"I'm killing two birds at once, so to speak.
Animal-based food kills people.
This way, by going vegan...
we get healthy and save animals.
I'm being selfish, too, because if
I can get my employees healthier,
we cut down on sick days
and gain more productivity."
- Steve Wynn

"Running has the power to change your life.
It will make you fitter, healthier, even happier."
- Selene Yeager

"Education NOT Medication!"
- Robert O. Young

"Exercise your freedom to make healthy choices
and to take back your health."
- Robert O. Young

"Grow what you eat and eat what you grow."
- Robert O. Young

"Health care NOT Sick care!"
- Robert O. Young

"It's no big secret that an alkaline lifestyle can do wonders
- from helping you lose weight and making sure you stay healthy.
The alkaline diet is so effective that
even celebrities have committed to it."
- Robert O. Young

"Once you know and believe that over-acidity
causes every disease and most dis-ease,
then to ignore that fact is a form of suicide.
When you eat poorly,
you pull the trigger every day of your life,
and eventually the gun fires.
The bullet might hit you square in the head
like a massive heart attack,
or it may kill you more slowly like a cancer,
or it may simply put you in a fog for the next
15 years like Alzheimer's or dementia."
- Robert O. Young

"The blood never lies."
- Robert O. Young

"The body runs on electrons NOT calories."
- Robert O. Young

"The fish is only as healthy as the water it swims in.
If the water is clean YOU DO NOT GET SICK!"
- Robert O. Young

"Action conquers fear."
- Pete Zarlenga

"We all know how important eating breakfast is,
but a lot of us neglect it."
- Adam Zickerman

"A cancer diagnosis changes you forever and
you remember the exact moment you heard those words.
How you react and move forward is up to YOU"
- unknown

"A good laugh and a long sleep are
the best cures in the doctor's book."
- unknown

"Always remember that your present situation
is not your final destination.
The best is yet to come."
- unknown

"An apple a day keeps the doctor away!"
- unknown

"At any given moment you have the power to say
this is NOT how the story is going to end."
- unknown

"At the timberline where the storms strike with the most fury,
the sturdiest trees are found."
- unknown

"Cancer is a word, not a sentence."
- unknown

"Cancer puts you to the test and it also brings out the best in you."
- unknown

"Cancer may have started the fight, but I will finish it."
- unknown

"Do not give up, the beginning is always the hardest."
- unknown

"Every tomorrow has two handles.
We can take hold of it by the handle of anxiety,
or by the handle of faith."
-unknown

"Faith is daring to go beyond what the eyes can see."
- unknown

"Feed your faith and your fears will starve to death."
- unknown

"He who fears something gives it power over him."
- unknown

"He who takes medicine and neglects to diet
wastes the skill of his doctors."
- unknown

"Hope is a reality to keep the faith
that you will survive and be alive!"
- unknown

"Hope is the physician of each misery."
- unknown

"Hope sees the invisible, feels the intangible
and achieves the impossible."
- unknown

"It isn't our position but our disposition which makes us happy."
-unknown

"Life is like the ocean.
It can be calm or still,
and rough or rigid, but in the end,
it is always beautiful."
- unknown

"Life is not waiting for the storm to pass
- but go out and play in the rain!
Thank God for everything -
never, never, never forget you are loved."
- unknown

"Listening is loving."
- unknown

"Live to win!"
- unknown

"Look to this day, for it is life.
For yesterday is already a dream and tomorrow is only a vision.
But today well lived makes every yesterday a dream of happiness,
and every tomorrow a vision of hope."
- unknown

"Never give up HOPE!"
- unknown

"Never give up
Life is worth living
There is life after cancer."
- unknown

"Physical strength is measured by what we can carry;
spiritual by what we can bear."
-unknown

"Some see a hopeless end,
while others see an endless hope."
-unknown

"Sometimes you have to go through things
and not around them."
- unknown

"Survivors Day helps me suck
up the positives from others."
- unknown

"This too shall pass."
- unknown

"True healthcare reform starts in your kitchen,
not in Washington."
- unknown

"We cannot direct the wind but we can adjust the sails."
- unknown

"What Cancer Cannot Do,
Cancer is so limited...
- It cannot cripple LOVE - It cannot shatter HOPE
- It cannot corrode FAITH - It cannot destroy PEACE
- It cannot kill FRIENDSHIP - It cannot suppress MEMORIES
- It cannot silence COURAGE - It cannot invade the SOUL
- It cannot steal eternal LIFE - It cannot conquer the SPIRIT."
- unknown

"What lies behind us and what lies before us
are tiny matters compared to what lies within us."
- unknown

"You are NOT alone,
There are now millions of us!"
- unknown

"You can't smooth out the surf,
but you can learn to ride the waves."
- unknown

"You go through loss, anger, depression and
eventually you discover hope.
To share this discovery that's the best thing.
It puts value and meaning to the diagnosis."
- unknown

"You have to figure out your own way to deal with this diagnosis.
You learn about yourself, what you are made of.
This can be extraordinary and you want to share this,
help others who go through the same thing."
- unknown

"You're not dying from cancer - you're living with it!"
- unknown

Epilogue

You may be surprised about the people and/or quotes that were missing from this book. Part of the reason was to keep the book fairly short and also so the <u>end</u> of this book could be the <u>beginning</u> for you to keep reading even more inspiring and thought provoking quotes. Perhaps you start your own collection of quotes that have a personal meaning and inspire YOU? You'll also notice a few quotes from yours truly. Why not share a few thoughts or ideas I came up with and plant the seed that YOU too have probably at one time or another come up with some profound thoughts of your own? Why should other people be the only ones who come up with quotes? The next time you come up with a clever thought or saying, write it down and put some quotation marks around that idea or thought. Then share YOUR new quote with other people! If you come up with any really great quotes, please share them with us and we just might add them to one of our next books!

100% TOTAL SATISFACTION GUARANTEE:

If for ANY reason you are not 100% satisfied with the book, audio CD or DVD you purchased, just send the product back along with receipt (or proof of payment). We will gladly refund 100% of your money, no questions asked!

Nemours Marketing, Inc.
7531 Azurebrook Court
Winter Park, FL 32792
info@NemoursMarketing.com
Tel: (407) 738 - 1608

www.ingramcontent.com/pod-product-compliance
Lightning Source LLC
Chambersburg PA
CBHW060308290526
45789CB00001B/445